Overwhelmed & Undernourished:

Use Food as Medicine and Turn Your Life Around

By Karen Thomas

January 2016

Overwhelmed & Undernourished:
Use Food as Medicine and Turn Your Life Around

Published by Holistic Digestive Solutions
Copyright © 2016 by Karen Thomas

Editing by Paula High

For permission requests, email the publisher or author at
karen@holisticdigestivesolutions.com

To contact the author, visit www.holisticdigestivesolutions.com

Bio-IINdividuality™, Institute for Integrative Nutrition®, Integrative Nutrition®, and IIN® trademarks owned by Integrative Nutrition, Inc. (used with permission).

Circle of Life, Primary Food(s), and Secondary Food(s): © 2005 Integrative Nutrition, Inc. (used with permission).

Functional Diagnostic Nutrition® and D.R.E.S.S for Health Success® are registered trademarks of Functional Diagnostic Nutrition® and FDN, Inc.

ISBN-10: 0-9968625-0-1
ISBN-13: 978-0-9968625-0-9

Library of Congress Control Number: 2016905810
Holistic Digestive Solutions, Raleigh, NC 27613

Printed in the United States of America

Table of Contents

---

[1] The Circle of Life: ©2005 Integrative Nutrition, Inc. (used with permission).

Dedication

I dedicate this to my husband, Jimmy, for whom I am forever grateful. I don't deserve you but I am ecstatic that God placed you in my life. Thank you!

I also dedicate this to my mom, Josefa Mori, from whom I gain my strength. It is because of you that I made it through the amazingly difficult time. Thanks for praying for me and being my biggest cheerleader.

And I dedicate this to all the sick people out there. I've been sick too, and I understand much of your struggle. I did this for you, so you don't have to stay sick anymore.

Acknowledgements

My heartfelt thanks to the following people:

My family, who prayed for me during these last few years, even though I hid the depths of depression from them. Thank you all.

Monika Miles, my college roommate and friend. Thanks for calling me every day to check-in on me, while I was sick. You demonstrated true friendship and I'm so grateful for you.

Monica Scudieri gave me some marvelous advice during the time I needed it most: "Since you're unable to work, find a way to get up, out of bed, and go to the bookstore. Start reading on thyroid conditions. Read, Read, Read." When I followed your advice, I could not believe what I learned. Thanks!

Pastor Dick VanCleave, (Ret.) RFA – Elder, my pastoral counselor at Raleigh First Assembly of God. You were the only person I truly felt safe talking to when I was so sick. I felt I could count on you to be truthful with me, no matter what. You prayed for me and with me. Thank you so much for your guidance. I'm eternally grateful for your counsel, and I wish I could still see you.

Peggie D'Amico, from Raleigh First Assembly of God. Thank you for filling out paper work for me, when I wasn't able to think or write for myself.

Leah A. Carmo, MEd, MS, LMHC, my dear friend who saved my life twice. It took Leah all of 15 seconds hearing how sick I'd been, to tell me about a neurotransmitter test she could run on me. You finally figured out exactly what was going on in my brain and affecting my body. Thanks a million.

Diane Hemmer, whose profound words saved me years of counseling. During our conversation about family dynamics, she hit the nail on the head, allowing me more healing. Thank you for the illumination about issues that were never mine to carry. It's a relief to finally understand, there was nothing "wrong with me," and I did nothing to incur the burden. Thanks for your words of wisdom.

To my Institute for Integrative Nutrition® friends: For all my IIN® friends who inspired me to write this book. Thanks for your encouragement and pushing to really make it happen.

To Melissa Vance, my accountability partner through our education at Institute for Integrative Nutrition®. Thank you for listening to me and keeping me accountable. Thanks for your concern while I tried different protocols to get my health back and for letting me cry every time I needed to.

Tremendous thanks to Paula High, not only my classmate, friend, and colleague, but someone who also brought me her distinctive magic as an editor and book doctor. I'm grateful for the opportunity to practice on you. Thanks for taking my deepest thoughts, fixing, rearranging, and clarifying them. You helped bring the dream of my book to life.

Patricia Smith Wood, thank you for lending your assistance as a third set of eyes. Your double and triple checking of the manuscript was invaluable. Your professional guidance, as an editor and a published author, is appreciated beyond words.

Joe Cross, thank you so very much for bringing your documentary, *Fat, Sick and Nearly Dead* to the masses. Without it, I might have done the unthinkable: give up and permanently check out of this wonderful life. Because you developed the Juicing Boot Camp, I learned about the importance of whole foods for healing.

Natalie Lowell, I'm so glad you were my boot camp coach. You saw me through that time and know how my life has been changed—thanks to your help and truly healthy food.

Thanks to my boot camp group, for allowing me to share my deepest pain, when I felt little hope. You all supported me and showed you understood. I'm glad some of us still stay in contact. You're the best!

Ajana Lima, I thank you for helping me with proof reading and design input.

Jennifer Ellis-Schuetz, FDN-P, thank you for the terrific description of chronic fatigue.

Reed Davis, CNT, FDN Founder, thank you for the informative course you offer, and for helping me in supporting and promoting this book.

Brandon Mollé, from Functional Diagnostic Nutrition®, I thank you for all your help with the few last minute tweaks of information and your clarifications.

Dr. Henry VanPala, MD, thank you for your ongoing support and for agreeing to contribute to the Foreword in this book.

And finally—Joshua Rosenthal, thank you (times 1000) for developing the Institute for Integrative Nutrition® and pouring your heart and soul into it. Your love and wisdom shines through every module. Because the Institute has become so popular and well-respected, I discovered it and sign on for one of the best experiences of my life. I'm delighted you included many of the best speakers in the holistic and integrative wellness movement.

May God bless you all.

Praise for Karen Thomas and Overwhelmed & Undernourished

"Karen Thomas, author of *Overwhelmed & Undernourished: Use Food as Medicine and Turn Your Life Around*, is a graduate of the Institute for Integrative Nutrition® (IIN®). At IIN®, she completed a cutting edge curriculum in nutrition and health coaching taught by the world's leading experts in health and wellness. I recommend you read this book and get in touch with Karen to see how she can help you successfully achieve your goals."

– Joshua Rosenthal, MScEd, Founder/Director, Institute for Integrative Nutrition®

"Ms. Karen Thomas has pulled together a remarkably helpful and informative book with a fascinating and heartwarming personal saga. Her motivational message, looks at real answers to common health predicaments. For all who have struggled with personal and family health problems, Karen's story of trials, tribulations, and triumphs will lift you up as she shares her discoveries, and preserves her convictions."

– Reed Davis, Founder, Functional Diagnostic Nutrition® Certification Course

Foreword

by Dr. Henry VanPala, MD

"If I had it to do all over again, what would I do differently?"

If you've ever asked yourself this question, Karen Thomas is able to give you the answer to that and more, in her book *Overwhelmed & Undernourished: Use Food as Medicine and Turn Your Life Around.*

I first met Karen as a patient in my gastroenterology practice, in 2014. At that time, she had already traveled on a long and arduous journey, seeking solutions to various physical problems. I have observed her amazing transformation into total health and wellness. I am in awe of her persistence in gaining knowledge. Her perseverance and understanding of today's health issues helps her utilize this knowledge in her everyday life.

I'm so confident in Karen's knowledge of nutrition and food-related illness, that I often refer my own patients to her. She taught me more about nutrition than I learned as a board-certified, Yale trained gastroenterologist. More than 30 years after recertification in both gastroenterology and internal medicine, what I knew about food hadn't changed. I now realize that the intestinal microbiome—the millions of bacteria that inhabit the intestine from the stomach to the anus—is thought to be the most important aspect of maintaining a healthy life. It is also one of the main determinants for disease.

The intestinal microbiome has far reaching importance—from simple things like food allergies, regulatory hormones, inflammatory responses—all the way to recognizing determinants of developing certain cancers. This bacterial environment affects how people feel every day. Even common things like bloating, irritable bowel syndrome, and inflammatory diseases such as ulcerative colitis or Crohn's disease, are linked to the intestinal microbiome.

It has been definitively proven that the bacteria in your intestines determines whether you will be a fat person or a thin one. With the world's increasing obesity epidemic, this issue is one of the most important risk factors for cancer, heart disease, diabetes, and multiple other health problems.

Understanding the importance of the intestinal microbiota, perhaps the entire medical field needs to embrace learning the importance of food in regulating our daily and future health.

Overwhelmed & Undernourished tells the story of Karen's stressful journey over the course of several years. It relates her strength in taking over her situation. You'll learn the steps she finally took to regain complete health. Her determination to understand the root cause of her steep decline led her to investigate the broad field of nutrition. That led to her study of Integrative Nutrition® and Functional Diagnostic Nutrition®. Her successful completion of the IIN® coursework qualifies her to share her knowledge. To people suffering from chronic fatigue, fibromyalgia, leaky gut, celiac disease, migraines, weight loss resistance, and much more—this book offers a ray of hope and a path to success.

-Henry Joseph VanPala, MD, RPh, AGA
North Hills Internal & Integrative Medicine, PA
Board Certified Internal Medicine, 1984, 2010
Board Certified Gastroenterology, 2013
Board Certified Obesity, 2016
Raleigh, North Carolina

* * *

Introduction

This book was written for the many people in the country today who find themselves in a situation similar to what Karen Thomas experienced in 2012. While it is the particular story of one person's journey from debilitating illness to recovering health, her path may not be common to everyone. However, in today's world of fast, processed and genetically modified foods, almost anyone can find themselves feeling tired, puffy, and lethargic. For those people and many others like them, this book is an inspiration. The solutions for so many illnesses can be found in learning proper nutrition and being open to functional and integrative healthcare.

Fortunately, today's patients have more and better tools to aid in their recovery. It can be as simple as changing your food habits, and learning what helps your body and what harms it. Integrative and functional medicine is coming into it's own as it shows people how to alleviate illness, using natural whole foods and supplements, rather than continuing down the path of pharmaceuticals and harmful toxins.

If reading Karen's story inspires you to investigate the modalities she used to regain her health, she has fulfilled one of her dreams—helping other people like her back to health and happiness.

Paula High, BS, Communications;
Integrative Nutrition® Health Coach;
Herbalist; Essential Oils Educator;
Writer and Editor

Patricia Smith Wood, Author,
The Easter Egg Murder,
Murder on Sagebrush Lane
Editor, Teramar Corporation

Chapter 1

The Perfect Storm

Stress Kills

YOU'VE PROBABLY HEARD the phrase, "stress kills." But I never knew how true it was, until I went through my own struggles with it. A few little life changes, here and there, seemed like normal stuff. I figured one by one, I'd tackle them—no problem. But one by one—and another one—and another one, and . . . Never could I have imagined what was about to happen to me, and how it would change my life forever.

Graduating School and Preparing for a New Career

Who knew what monster was lurking, just around the corner in my seemingly calm life. I knew things were about to change a little. In 2005, I finished my bachelor's degree in Dental Hygiene, at University of North Carolina. That meant a nice career change in the coming months and a better income, which was scary and exciting. However, the monster stalking me was sneaky, quiet, and formidable. I was completely unprepared for the attack.

While finishing my degree, I noticed hives breaking out on my skin. I chalked it up to the stress of finals, graduation, and upcoming job changes. No big deal, right? I figured it would go away. So of course I didn't clue-in. I ignored it. But it was the dawn of the scariest time of my life. This little symptom was the beginning of many physiological changes in my body.

1

As 2005 passed, I kept on working full time in my old job as a clinical hygienist and going to school in the evenings, preparing to graduate. When I finally went to a doctor about the hives, I was diagnosed with urticaria[2] (hives).

I had experienced hives before. Lots of people get them. They're fairly common, but I had no idea it was my body telling me, "Wake up and pay attention—something is going on! Something is wrong!" Maybe I should have figured this out long ago. Every time I was under stress, I developed hives the size of my hands, all over my body. But I didn't "connect the dots."

Stress Levels

It is fairly well known that life events and changes are among the most common forms of stress. A few of the more stressful events are: changing jobs, getting married, getting divorced, losing a spouse, death in the family, moving to a new location, or having a baby. By looking at a list of those you've experienced in the last year or two, you can gauge how high or low your stress level has been. But it can become debilitating when those events start piling up, and chaos breaks loose in your life.

A New Career

One of the first changes in my life, around that time, was a new job. In 2006, I went from being a clinical dental hygienist, into the world of research. It was a whole new arena of information and circumstances to take in. Learning a new job was stressful enough, but I had added another life event: I got engaged a couple of months prior to the new job. I started planning our wedding. I seemed to be a glutton for punishment. It's as if I were thinking, *"Pile it on please. Can I have more?"*

Meet the Fiancée

Jimmy, my fiancée, worked full time as a Program Engineer at IBM. I'd known him for several years as one of my dental

---

[2] Urticaria is the medical name for hives.

patients. In 2003 he became divorced and asked me for my phone number. At first, I didn't take him seriously. I figured he was just another guy hitting on me. I quietly sent out a request to God—if this was meant to be, Jimmy would ask again for my number. Within a minute, he repeated his request. I acted like I was ignoring him—until he left. Then I gave him the piece of paper with my number on it. We dated for three and a half years, before he proposed, in 2005.

Illness Within the Family

While events were stacking up in my life, my future mother-in-law became very ill. It was difficult for all of us. We spent the next eight months with her, in and out of the hospital. It was hard not knowing, from one day to the next, if her health would improve or decline. We were desperately hoping she would be well enough to make it to the wedding. Jimmy was the first of all her children to get married in the Church. God and Church were very important to her. So we navigated through that time, anxiously waiting, hoping and praying she would rally and be able to attend.

Searching for, and Buying Our New Home-Sweet-Home

In addition to all I've mentioned so far, Jimmy and I decided to buy a house together, near the Raleigh, NC area. Since we each already had homes of our own; we planned to sell them and find a house to meet both our needs. We had to answer the big question: how do you bring together, in one house, the country-living guy, and city girl?

This was no easy task. I had my list of must-haves, and he had his. But guess what? In September 2006, we finally found a house—with the right potential. Easy you think? Not so much. What we found was a house in the country with acreage to meet his needs, and a large kitchen to meet mine.

Great, you'd think. But Wait! There's More! We found a house that was only eight years old but reminded me of that scary,

Herman Munster house from television.[3] It looked like it had been abandon for years, and possibly haunted. It was so bad, people would drive by this house and ask the neighbors what happened to it.

I still remember calling my mom and saying, "We found a house, but it's a piece of crap."

She gave me what I'm sure seemed like great advice—because she couldn't imagine how bad it was. "Let him do what he wants. He can fix it up and make it better."

Until she saw it . . . . By then, it was too late. She asked, "Oh my. Couldn't you take a bulldozer, plow it down, and start all over?"

"No Mom, we can't."

I wished it were possible. It might have been so much easier.

At this point, we'd already sold Jimmy's house. The proceeds would go toward remodeling the new house. So we decided to keep mine, since the "new" house needed so much work. We had just bought all new furniture, so we chose to keep it in my house. That way it wouldn't be destroyed while we cleaned and worked on the "new" one.

To illustrate how bad it was, it took two professional cleaners, two full days, to clean the inside of our new house. After that, I spent another 30 days cleaning just the kitchen. I remember how awful it was spending all day, every day, for a month, cleaning that nasty kitchen. It was SO gross.

One weekend, I decided to stay in the house. I worked until 10 pm or later, and then planned to take a shower and start all over again in the morning. I got ready for my first shower in the house. I turned on the water, and it dripped! *What? A drip? No water pressure? Are you kidding me? What is going on?*

---

[3] Herman Munster was a character on an American television comedy called, *The Munster's*, in the mid-1960s, on the CBS network. The Munsters were a creepy, ghoulish family living in a scary house.

I called Jimmy. In his repair attempts, he broke a piece of the shower faucet, making things worse. When I looked up at the ceiling, what did I see? Roaches! UGH! The entire house was apparently infested with the awful creatures.

By then, I was crying, and thought—*what has this man done to me? Does he not understand? I will not be able to live through this. I cannot live in a place that has bugs or needs major construction.*

But it was too late for that. I had to suck it up and deal with it. This was only the beginning of our adventures in this house. My downward spiral into depression had begun, but I was in denial about it for quite some time.

After a few months, I'd grown to hate the house, but what could I do? I kept on planning our wedding. I continued going back and forth to the hospital, at all hours of the day and night, for my future mother-in-law. Ah. But at least I still had a *clean, safe* haven to go to—my "other" house.

The Wedding

A week before our April wedding, my mother-in-law had her first stroke. With only seven days before the wedding, our prayer was, "God, please keep her alive so she can come to our wedding, and see her son married in the Church."

She was in the hospital the day of our wedding in April 2007, but the doctors allowed her out long enough to attend. At the reception, she passed out and everyone initially thought she had *died*. We took her back to the hospital, and the cycle of stroke and heart issues continued.

SUMMARY: *Just to keep score for you—It was spring 2007, I was now married with a house under major construction, working full-time (in a new career), and dealing with a sick mother-in-law. I had a few months with things as they were. It was tough, but I figured it couldn't get much worse. It did.*

Going Down in Flames

Things were hard, but we were plugging along. Surely life as I knew it, couldn't possibly get any worse. Oh why did I have to say that? Of course it could, and *did*.

Thinking I was maxed out on all possible stressors, I received a phone call. It was "The Ides of March," (3/15/08). This time, my house was on fire. *(Oh, is that all?)* Of course I asked which one. I was secretly hoping it was the "new" house, which was under major construction.

Nope. Of course not. That would be so mundane. It was MY house—the house in which all our brand new furniture was sitting. Gone. My refuge from the nastiness and construction, and the place I would go to hide from the world. It was my one nice, spotless home—the place I could still call my sanctuary. There, I could escape, be alone and cry. Now it was gone.

My house had taken an indirect lightning strike. It struck between my house and my neighbor's house. The current caught my phone line, traveled around and up through my garage and back down. It ignited under the house, in the crawl space. How it didn't completely burn to the ground was a miracle. But it was a total loss inside. It had to be gutted to be repaired.

The insurance company took over contracting out the repairs. It was like a giant game of "Jenga®,"[4] as they braced flooring and walls to replace floor joists, while not collapsing the entire structure. The whole interior of my house had to be gutted. The floors, ceilings, walls, all cabinets, and even the toilets had to be replaced. It was unlivable.

Now I had a blue Porta Potty to visit, for the next year. Yes, it took one entire year to rebuild, into 2009. Oh yeah, I almost

---

[4] Jenga® is a tumbling-tower, blocks game of balance & strategy. First developed by Leslie Scott in the early 1970s, licensing eventually landed at Hasbro's Parker Brothers division by the mid '80s. https://en.wikipedia.org/wiki/Jenga

forgot to mention. When this happened, a buyer was planning to fly in the next day to sign the papers to buy my house.

At this point, we had to move into the *new* home, even though it was a major construction zone and work in progress. You already know how unpopular this was with me. I now had two houses under construction. Our new, work-zone home and mine, which stunk so badly of smoke and toxic, melted materials that I had to completely change clothes when I got *home* . . . to our new home. My house smelled awful for many months, until renovations finally, gradually removed the stench.

By then, I felt something had to give. I was thinking, *I should just admit myself into the psych-ward at the hospital. I do work near a hospital; so it would be handy . . . just a walk next door and I'd be there. Oh wait. No, it's too close to work. They might still have me working, between therapy groups. So what would be the point? Never mind.*

Death in the Family

A few months later, in October of 2008, I remember getting a phone call from the New York State Police Department. They asked me who Dennis Ryan was, because they found my phone number on the back of his driver's license.

"That's my dad," I responded. He was actually my stepfather, but he was dad to me.

They said I needed to get to the hospital, in New York. What happened? The short version: My dad was on his way to work, and he died. The Police had gone to my parent's house but my mom was out running errands. So I had to find my mom and tell her and my brother the sad news. Jimmy and I flew up to New York and helped her with all the arrangements.

SUMMARY: *October 2008: Newly married with two houses under major construction; no refuge to escape to; grieving the loss of my beautiful, clean, sanctuary home; working full-time in a new career; still dealing with a sick mother-in-law in and out of the*

7

hospital; seriously over-tired; grieving over the loss of my dad; I needed time to grieve, but there was barely time to breathe.

I experienced so much guilt over not being able to help my mom as much as I felt I should; not being able to SEE her and give her the support I wanted to give her.

I asked for time off from work, but they wouldn't give it to me. At this point I should have made some changes, but no. I continued on like a trooper. I was obviously still in denial about the depression plaguing me. I thought I could do it all, mostly because I thought it couldn't get any worse. But . . . It did!!

Really? How much worse could this get? Seriously? STOP!! As if I was done. Ha!

Chapter 2

The Storm Intensified

JUST UNDER A year passed. Jimmy continued working on our "new" house throughout everything. His usual routine was to leave work around 3:00 pm and immediately resume the remodeling upon getting home. He usually worked on the construction until about 11:00 pm. Then he collapsed into bed.

By spring of 2009, it was about two-thirds of the way complete. It was great to have the progress coming along. But I was secretly mad at him for spending all his time working on the house. I felt a bit neglected. I suppose it might have been the depression I wasn't yet admitting to feeling.

That same spring, I finally sold my house, as reconstruction was wrapping up. The proceeds from selling my house went toward further remodeling on the "new" house, paying off my student loans, and other bills. I kept working full time through everything, as well.

New Husband Needs Major Warranty Work

A few months later, at the end of May 2009, I decided to give my sister-in-law, Ana, a surprise baby shower. I finally had something upbeat to look forward to—my first nephew

I live in North Carolina, but she lived in Florida at the time. She worked in a restaurant. I called her boss to enlist his assistance. As planned, Ana's boss called her into work on her day off. We showed up at her job, and "SURPRISE!" There we were, bearing gifts for our new bundle of joy. It was successful, and we were all excited for the new life we were welcoming.

The next day, I made a phone call to check on my husband. He was fine when I left, but he has a 20-year history of deep vein thrombosis (DVT's)[5]. So I tend to worry a bit. When he didn't answer, I thought it was strange. Since I was duly concerned, I called my other sister-in-law Kay, my husband's sister.

"Where's my husband?" I sternly inquired, once she answered her mobile phone.

"Well, I don't want you to yell at him, but he had a headache last night, and he passed out. But he's OK now."

"Let me talk to him please."

Turns out they had gone to the beach for the weekend. When I talked to him, I could tell it was not good.

I thought, *Geeze, with his blood issue history, why the hell didn't they call 911?*

And there I was, stuck in Florida while he was ill in North Carolina. I asked my family to pray for him, because I knew it was bad, and I couldn't get home on an earlier flight.

He seemed OK on the surface, but I knew better. Jimmy drove home from the beach, back to Raleigh, and then picked me up at the airport. He told me he made an appointment with the doctor for later that day. I was grateful, because he was going, no matter what.

The funny thing is, he asked me if I would wait in the car while he went into his appointment. I laughed.

---

[5] DVT or deep vein thrombosis is a blood clotting disorder.

"What you're telling me is—if I were sick and went into see the doctor, and I asked you to wait in the car—you would actually do that?"

He grinned sheepishly, "Well, yeah,"

"Really? Well, guess what? I'm not you, and I will be going in with you."

We arrived in his doctor's office and went into the exam room. The doctor came in and Jimmy explained what had happened. She told Jimmy he is not the normal, average patient. He has a blood disorder and needs to take *everything* that happens to him very seriously.

After the exam, she was visibly frustrated. "It's been too long since the incident occurred, so I'm not sure what to do."

If only you knew me, you'd already know this didn't sit well with me. With all the other stuff going on, I don't know how I was able to think. *I knew* what needed to happen. I am grateful God was with me, guiding me.

I calmly advised the doctor, "OK, this is what you are going to do. I want you to order a CAT Scan. I don't care where the testing location is or what time. I want to see what is going on in his brain."

Deep down, when I'd spoken to Jimmy on the phone, I already had a feeling of what was wrong. She agreed and started the process. When Jimmy stood from the exam table, the nurse noticed he was unstable. The medical term is "ataxia." She called the doctor back in.

Jimmy is so funny. He made the proverbial "muscle pose" implying, "See I'm strong."

I was thinking, *Really? Oh please.* The doctor left the room and made some adjustments to the chart.

I later found out, they usually call 911 for visits like Jimmy's. That's because typically, once the husband gets in the car, he tells the wife, "I'm not going to any damned hospital."

They knew me well enough, so they had no problem letting me take him across the street to the hospital. They already knew I wouldn't let him talk me out of going.

When we arrived at the hospital for his CAT Scan, I called his sister. I asked her to come stay there with him, while I went back to the airport, to retrieve my luggage. In all the chaos, I hadn't had time to pick it up at the baggage claim after getting off my flight home.

The next bit of news came by way of yet another dreaded phone call. (I don't even know why I still had a phone anymore. It *always* seemed to be bad news!) The hospital called to tell me Jimmy had a "cerebral hematoma"—his brain was bleeding. They were admitting him to the ICU to watch him.

After a few days in ICU (it was early June 2009, by this time), they decided to send him home. When I got him home, I realized that something was still seriously wrong. He couldn't walk by himself from the car to the couch.

My mom happened to call me at that point. She asked, "Do you want me to come."

I didn't want to bother her, but told her, "Yes please."

As soon as I got off the phone with her, I logged into the computer and booked her flight for the next day. Thank God for moms. I would not have made it through this, if it weren't for her strength and wisdom.

The next day, my mom arrived and Jimmy, was not getting any better. I called the neurosurgeon and told him something was still wrong with Jimmy. The doctor told me to get him to the hospital, and he would order another CAT Scan.

Emergency Neurosurgery

When we got there, I called the neurosurgeon again. I told him Jimmy was in the CT machine, and he should look on his computer immediately to see what the CAT Scan was showing, because something was wrong.

I waited on the phone while the doctor looked at the scan. He told me get to his office right away. Thank God it was next door!

Once we had Jimmy in the doctor's office, they told us he had so much blood on his brain that it was shifting. The doctor said, "We are going to do surgery this afternoon."

Jimmy decided he needed to use the bathroom. On the way to the restroom, a few steps away, he passed out. My mom and I caught him, and the doctor said, "Let's get him to the hospital and do the surgery now!"

Back at the hospital once again, the surgery prep process began. They shaved half his head, and off he went into surgery. My entire family had gathered by then, and waited with me in the ICU waiting room.

The waiting was difficult, but he made it through the surgery. I was first to see him. I entered the recovery room, and Jimmy looked at me and then at the nurse. He looked back at me quizzically, "Who is this person?"

Thank God I know my husband's twisted humor. I looked at the nurse and then at Jimmy, "I see she is very pretty. Are you showing off?"

I told the nurse she would enjoy having him as one of her patients, because he has a sense of humor and a great attitude. He laughed. I don't know how all of this didn't completely derail me, with all the stress I was feeling, but somehow I kept going.

They took him back to his room in ICU. I told the family they could go see him, but not to be thrown if he claimed not to recognize them. He *is* a practical joker.

This turned out to be the easy part. All of this had been scary enough. Little did I know it at the time, but we were only getting started with Jimmy's hospital adventure. What was about to happen was going to *blow my mind*. It would test me and stretch me to my limits.

Chapter 3

Rocking the Boat

Who's Really in Charge?

AT SOME POINT in June 2009, I finally realized I had no true control over what was happening. I felt like I couldn't take on any more stress. It reminded me of Job, in the bible.

I was so stressed I couldn't even cry anymore. My heart had become like a rock. I was drained and had no more emotions. I felt dead inside. I was just going day by day, until all of the hell would stop. I felt like I had lived 50 years' worth of stress, in just a few months. I could not do it anymore. I was about to break. And yet, I was still in denial about the depression.

I felt like saying, "Hey Jimmy, maybe we can move another bed into your hospital room, and I can have a break-down while you get your treatment."

How Could Things Get Any Worse?

I always felt like summer was supposed to be a fun time. This had not been a fun summer. In July 2009, they sent Jimmy home. I was glad to finally have him come home. The schedule had been grueling. I was exhausted. I had not been able to take any time off. I continued working. I saw my patients in the mornings and then left for the hospital, to see Jimmy in ICU, until around 8:00

pm each night. Then I drove home to return phone calls and let everyone know how he was doing. I woke up at 5:00 am the next morning. Back to the same weird routine. By the way, did I mention I couldn't get any decent sleep either?

Back Home

When I brought Jimmy home, again, I knew something still wasn't right. I sensed I would have to watch him that first night home, but I wasn't sure how. I needed sleep. I felt completely drained: physically, mentally, and emotionally. I couldn't even think. I could barely move or function.

I prayed to Jesus, "Please help me just get through this night."

The next thing I knew, it was Sunday morning and Jimmy got up to take a shower, while I lay in bed. I suspected once I got up, the peace would be over. I had an uneasy feeling about what was coming.

During the night, I'd heard Jimmy's labored breathing. I asked him about it, but he told me it was normal, and he was just tired. I knew deep inside; this next day was going to be *one of those days*.

When he came out of the bathroom, he passed out, barely missing his head, near his surgery scar. I screamed for my mom, grabbed the phone, and called 911. As I spoke with the 911 operator, my mom began to pray over Jimmy.

They asked me if he was breathing. I said, "No, he is turning gray."

I just wanted to get off the phone so I could start CPR. I told the operator I was positioning him to start rescue breathing and compressions, and to stop asking me questions. Thank God for my CPR training.

I became aware of hearing my mom calling Jimmy back from the dead, like Jesus called Lazarus back.

NIV, JOHN 11: 38-44
Jesus Raises Lazarus from the Dead

38 Jesus, once more deeply moved, came to the tomb. It was a cave with a stone laid across the entrance.

39 "Take away the stone," he said. "But, Lord," said Martha, the sister of the dead man, "by this time there is a bad odor, for he has been there four days."

40 Then Jesus said, "Did I not tell you that if you believe, you will see the glory of God?"

41 So they took away the stone. Then Jesus looked up and said, "Father, I thank you that you have heard me.

42 I knew that you always hear me, but I said this for the benefit of the people standing here, that they may believe that you sent me."

43 When he had said this, Jesus called in a loud voice, "Lazarus, come out!"

44 The dead man came out, his hands and feet wrapped with strips of linen, and a cloth around his face. Jesus said to them, "Take off the grave clothes and let him go."

Suddenly, I saw Jimmy breathing. A miracle, right before my eyes! The (EMS) emergency medical staff arrived. I told them to take him back to the same hospital where his neurosurgeon was. I told the EMS that I believed Jimmy had developed a blood clot, because he was taken off his blood thinners, due to the brain bleed and surgery.

I followed them to the hospital. When I was in the emergency room, the staff asked me, "What do you do for a living? You're surprisingly calm."

Amazingly, I *was* calm. I told them I worked in dentistry.

The on-call doctor informed us that Jimmy had blood clots from his ankles all the way up into his chest. They decided to put in an IVC filter (inferior vena cava filter). It would only help any clots which formed in his extremities. They could only watch any clots in his chest. Jimmy was admitted back into ICU, and we prayed for the best.

Once out of his procedure, I met Jimmy back in his room. Of course the doctors were surprised to see him, yet again. They decided to keep him for observation for a while. The blood clots in his legs were expected to be OK, since he had a filter. Those would go through the filter and dissolve. The clots in his chest, they hoped, would not move.

Since he'd just had surgery on his brain, they could not put him back on Coumadin, a blood thinner. This was problematic. They needed the blood clot on his brain to stay lodged where it was so he wouldn't bleed any more. If that particular clot did not remain in place, it would mean more surgery, and God knows what else.

The next bit of news, left me feeling like . . . well, like I just couldn't take anymore. The doctors told me Jimmy would have to be in ICU for the next six to eight weeks, and he would not be able to move, due to the clots in his chest and lungs.

Of course I was stoic, no tears allowed. No external hint of the chaos reigning inside. There was no time to cry. I had to be cool and stay in control, because I needed to think like a professional, not like a wife.

But Wait. There's More! "Please Make It Stop."

Sometimes it seems as if the intensive care unit doctors assume, since most of their patients in ICU are near death and can't speak, it's why they belong there. Because Jimmy could speak and joke around, they seemed to think he must not belong there anymore.

Within days, they went from saying he needed to be observed in ICU for eight weeks, to wanting to move him to another unit, on a different floor. My gut feeling was they were very wrong.

"No." I pleaded with them. "He is not ready for that. Just because he is able to speak, do not assume he is OK. He is *not* OK."

But they *did* move him to another unit, upstairs. I was flabbergasted. He was up there for less than eight hours, before trouble struck again. That evening, when he stood to go for a walk, he experienced a sudden shortness of breath. It was a sure sign one of the clots in his chest moved.

They had to put him on oxygen, and the next morning, they moved him back to ICU. I was so frustrated, but I kept praying and asking God for help. What happened next, was nothing short of another miracle.

A Room with Ventilation

The next day, (the end of July 2009) I was on my way back to the hospital to see Jimmy, when my phone rang again. I saw the number and felt the dread rising up from the pit of my stomach.

I answered and heard an urgent voice. "We need you to come to the hospital right away. We are trying to keep your husband alive. One of the blood clots in his chest moved into his heart, and he is on a ventilator. We are calling all over the country to see what we can do to keep him alive."

I went directly to the hospital, and what they told me should have completely devastated me, but somehow, it didn't.

The doctors told me, if they air lifted him to Duke Hospital and did thoracic surgery he would die. If they did surgery on him where he was, he would die. Basically, anything they might do would kill him. Period. They told me, "Go and say good-bye to your husband."

That's when I started talking to God again.

"God? Here is the deal. Jimmy belongs to you. He was yours first, and you have blessed me with him for this short time. I have no control over this situation."

I took a deep breath, steadied myself, and continued. "If you choose to take him home now, please know that I will always serve you. I will not be angry, because I know you love him more than I do. So I put him in your hands. If you choose to heal him and give him back to me, I will be so very happy and grateful. I give this to you, Lord."

Never before, in all my life, had I experienced the sense of peace and calm in my being, as I was in that moment. I think it was because I knew I had no control over any of it. Please understand, for a control freak like me, this was amazing. God was in control, not me. It was the best place to be.

I remembered Matthew 11:28:

"Come to me, all you who are weary and burdened, and I will give you rest."

Just then, one of the doctors came to me and told me the surgery they had decided to perform was very serious. I needed to say good-bye to my husband.

The first thing out of my mouth was, "I am a Christian and I believe God is in charge here."

This first doctor responded, "I too am a Christian."

"Well Praise God."

Apparently, since I was so calm and not crying, they thought I didn't "get it." They didn't understand what I was trying to tell them. A second doctor was sent in to talk with me.

"Do you understand how serious this surgery is?"

A little louder, and with more conviction I told him, "*I am a Christian.*"

Again, he didn't seem to understand my meaning. They all thought I was not getting the seriousness of the surgery. Yet again, they sent the next doctor in, with the same message.

"Do you understand how serious this is?"

At this point, I thought, *I told you I am a Christian, and I believe God is in charge here. What part of that do you guys not understand?* But they didn't truly understand my statement. They sent in the fifth doctor, or was it the sixth?

When I saw him coming toward me, I could see he was visibly shaking. He appeared to be the surgeon who would perform the surgery. *Great.*

He sternly said to me, "I know the other doctors have come in here and dropped the bomb of how serious this surgery is. We *need* you to *go* and say good-bye to your husband now."

By the end of his sentence, the doctor was practically yelling at me—as if it would shock me into *his* reality of Jimmy not making it through the surgery.

He clearly didn't comprehend how I could be so calm in the face of the situation, as he saw it. This seemed to frustrate him. I wanted to bring him into an understanding of how wrong, and truly tainted his thinking was—not just for Jimmy, but noxious to me, to my loved ones and, to the entire situation. How could he not see that his attitude was toxic?

Perhaps it's hard for some people to grasp the combination of feelings that were coursing through me that day. I experienced an intense, tranquil, glassy-smooth, yet steely calmness. It came from knowing that God and Holy Spirit were in charge there. Alongside that was an equally vigorous, firm, and absolute, faith—a conviction—that these doctors needed to accept the truth. They were not making the decision here. God was.

But I set him straight, and they *would* understand me.

In a fervent, passionate tone I spelled it out. "No! *You* don't get it. You don't understand. You are looking at things in the *world's* view. But *my* God is so much bigger than that. You must change your mindset. Now, go into the surgery with a positive attitude. You need to know—and grasp—that I am out here praying for you. God's anointing will come down from the Heavens, and it will go through my hands and *into yours*. Jimmy will be just fine."

The doctor left, still shaking and probably thinking, *"Wow this woman is a piece of work."* He had no idea what was about to happen, and how life-changing it would be for everyone to see.

It was standing room only in the operating area where Jimmy's procedure was performed. Due to the complexity of the surgery, it took them five hours. In those agonizingly long hours, the neurosurgeon came out several times to give me an update.

What I hadn't told most of the family, except for my mom and two others, was the doctors felt Jimmy wouldn't make it through. I decided I didn't want his family to be focused on the worst. I needed only positive thoughts, words, and people to be in the area.

The hours slowly passed. We could only imagine much of what was going on inside the surgery. My mom acted as the physical Holy Spirit for me. She recited scriptures from the Bible, having to do with faith, life, hope and happiness. Keeping the secret of what was really going on with Jimmy, I wanted to protect my spirit from any nonbelief.

Five hours after they began, the doctors came out and told me they couldn't believe how strong Jimmy was. I told them, "If you think he is strong, you need to meet my mother–in-law."

Then I asked, "OK, what's next?"

They told me they would move him to the recovery room, and then we could see him.

I couldn't believe my ears. It was like they were not thinking ahead. This was not acceptable.

So I corrected them. "Oh No! After what you've done to him, I need to know how much tPA [6] has been released into his brain.

"The CAT Scan machine is right here." I pointed and continued. "Please take a CAT Scan now, and then move him to recovery. That way, he can relax, and we can see what is going on in his brain now. Then we can get our next plan of action ready."

They looked at each other and then at me as if to say, "*Why didn't we already think about that?*" They did as I requested.

As they moved him from the CAT Scan room, the entire family lined the hallway to watch Jimmy go by. We did The WAVE as he passed us.

---

[6] tPA stands for tissue plasminogen activator, a blood clot buster medication.

His Talk with God

Not only did Jimmy survive the procedure, but he actually died five times and came back, while they were working on him. What helped him survive, was a conversation we recently had, while he was home on one of his hiatus days from the hospital.

Jimmy and I had a talk about what's important to God. I told him most people only ask for God's help when big things go wrong in their lives. But God wants everything, even the small stuff. I told him some people only pray when they need something substantial. But every detail is important to God, big and small.

Jimmy remembered this while he was in surgery. Every time they were losing him, he said it felt like an elephant was sitting on his chest. Then all of a sudden he had tremendous peace. Next, a light would appear and the light would get brighter and brighter. He then prayed.

The first time, he asked, "God, please let me stay. My mother is ill, and it isn't fair for a parent to have to bury one of her children."

Next, he heard the doctors say, "He's coming back."

The second time they started to lose him, he decided to pray for me. He said, "God, it isn't fair to make Karen a widow so soon after we just got married. Please let me stay with her."

Again, Jimmy heard the doctors, "He's coming back, he's coming back!"

It happened a few more times. The last time he said, "Well God, I have no one else to pray for, so if you are going to take me, then take me now."

Then he heard the doctors again, "We're done now, let's move him to recovery."

The next day, the doctors came and talked to him.

Jimmy said, "Thank God you guys had a pacemaker to help me come back."

They said, "No Jimmy. You don't understand. The pacemaker failed. It didn't work. You came back on your own."

This was God, our miracle worker. He answered my prayer. He gave Jimmy back to me.

Released, At Last

Finally, it was late July 2009, and Jimmy was released from the hospital again. I brought him home. By then, he could barely walk. He needed some physical rehabilitation, but I had to earn a living, even though I was completely exhausted. My mom helped nurse him back to health. They walked every day. They started with a few minutes a day, until they were walking three miles each day.

This left me time to go to work. I now realize what an idiot I was. With all the stress we had endured, and with all that was happening, I should have taken time off. But I didn't. I don't know what I thought I had to prove, except I believed I could handle it all.

And the Hits Just Keep on Coming

The day Jimmy was released from the hospital, my mother-in-law, Annie, went into the same hospital. She was in and out of there for the next few months. Annie struggled to get well. By January 2010, hospice was called in. Annie, unfortunately, was not able to get well. God took her home in April 2010.

If you think I was done with stressful situations at this time, you would be wrong. Jimmy was diagnosed with Melanoma. We buried Annie, and Jimmy had yet another surgery the day of her wake.

What Got Me Through the Entire Ordeal

Faith has always been an important part of my life. If it weren't for my faith in God, I can tell you things would have been so much more difficult for me.

Months before this crazy series of experiences happened to me, I had gone to church on one particular Sunday, at Raleigh First Assembly of God. I love my church. They had a speaker named Bishop June come in from Haiti. What I got from the sermon that day was burned deep into my spirit. He preached about a prophecy that was given to his father when he was born. He spoke about "The Promises of God." I know now why I was there that day. When I heard his message, I remembered it.

The summary of what his prophecy said to me that day was this:

If you get a promise from God and things don't look like they're going in that direction, put blinders on—like a horse. Do not look to the right, and do not look to the left. Keep your eyes focused on the Word of God. God's Word does not return void. It will come to pass, no matter what. God's Word does not lie. You just need to focus on the Word and believe, even if you don't see it.

The message soaked in for me. It told me when you are looking too closely at the situation, you stop looking at God's Word or Promise. When you've taken your eyes off His Word, you'll get derailed. Stay focused in the Word, and God's Word will stay in you.

That's what it meant for me, and I never forgot it. I remember God promising me things with Jimmy, my new husband. Losing him so soon was not what I remembered being the deal.

That's why I didn't tell Jimmy's family the entire, "truth," according to the doctors. I needed only strong believers to be around me, to encourage me when things didn't look good. Don't look to the right or the left, only at the Word of God. I remembered to keep my eyes on Jesus.

My mom has blessed me in so many ways, especially that day. She helped me keep it together. She let me lean on her, and she helped build me up in the waiting room. She whispered scriptures to me the entire time. I'm grateful for my mom and her tremendous faith. She loves me no matter what. She grounded herself in the Word of God and reminded me, minute by minute, who was really in charge.

I am forever grateful for the lessons I learned during this situation. Even when the ride gets bumpy, just hold on, because God will get you through this.

Chapter 4

The Downward Spiral Began

OK, A LOT has happened by this time and I'm sure it must be hard to keep track. So here's an instant replay for you.

2005: I graduated with my bachelor's degree, got engaged, and began a new career at the end of that year. 2006: Jimmy's mom was in and out of the hospital, and we bought that crazy house together. In 2007: Still dealing with Jimmy's mom being ill, and we got married.

In 2008 our new house was undergoing major remodeling, my house burned down, along with all of our new furniture, and then my father died.

About six months later, by spring of 2009, I was still working full-time and trying to manage all my grief, stress, and overwhelm. I was in denial about the depression. I finally sold *my* (newly rebuilt from fire damage) house. Remodeling continued on our new house, and by May 2009, it was about two-thirds finished.

Good thing, because that's when Jimmy landed in the hospital for a string of life-threatening issues. He was in and out of the hospital (mostly in) for three months. Jimmy was released in mid-summer of 2009. My mom had come to help out while

Jimmy was sick and recovering. All total, Jimmy was away from work for about six months, although everybody fought him on going back to work. Eventually, they compromised with a restricted, back-to-work agreement. But the work on the house was virtually at a stand-still for almost a year and a half. Just going to work every day was grueling enough for him. Plus, he was only allowed to lift a very small amount of weight. Everyone was hyper-concerned about anything he did. Jimmy couldn't really get back to the house remodeling until late 2010 or early 2011.

Denial

Meanwhile, those few years (2009-2013), I was on a slow decline, never taking time to notice the signs my body was showing me. Little by little, things started changing. There was an emotional and mental numbness running through me, and I couldn't process what was going on with my physical or mental state. I felt there was a disconnect between my brain and my body. I couldn't even cry.

Jimmy noticed various changes in me. "You do realize you're depressed, right?"

I still denied it, of course. For the longest time, I couldn't admit it. I couldn't see it, I couldn't feel it, and I was just . . . numb. Eventually I started realizing something was wrong—seriously wrong.

Work Schedule Shift

By spring 2012, I asked to change my work schedule from full-time, down to 30 hours per week. No one knew my dirty little secret. When I left my job Thursday afternoons, I was going home and sleeping, pretty much from Thursday afternoon until sometime Sunday. It gave me the partial recovery I needed to make it through my job Monday through Thursday. But I was declining at a faster rate than I was willing to admit. When the sleeping from Thursday to Sunday was not enough, I started feeling scared.

Sick and Tired, and zzzz . . .

One day I got off work at 4:00 pm. I remember calling Jimmy and telling him, "If you don't talk to me for my entire drive home, I will pull the car over and sleep right now."

I had never known this kind of exhaustion before. I've had conditions like pneumonia and Epstein Barr, and those were bad enough, but not like this. By late 2013, I had to withdraw from the job I had enjoyed so much, by taking medical leave. I was simply too sick to function.

I want you to understand how unbelievably debilitating something like this is. Had I not gone through it myself, I might not have believed it possible, other than hearing about it from time to time. Even then, I might have thought they were exaggerating. Indulge me as I try to sketch it out for you.

To describe chronic fatigue is difficult. It's not referring to the normal, average "tired" from everyday stressors or a long week. It's an intense kind of exhaustion, with a bizarre urgency to sleep immediately. It feels like if you can't curl-up somewhere to sleep, right away, you will just drop where you are and pass out.

A fellow Functional Diagnostic Nutrition® Practitioner (FDN-P)[7], Jennifer, explains chronic fatigue as ". . . feeling like you are running a marathon with a hangover, and the worst case of flu, all at the same time."

Each person who has endured it, probably has their own way of describing it. But I've yet to hear a description which truly does the experience justice.

One problem with disorders like chronic fatigue, depression or fibromyalgia, is you look fine on the outside, so no one believes you're ill. Since you don't have any physical evidence like a rash or a broken leg, people can't see it. There's a vague

---

[7] Functional Diagnostic Nutrition® is a registered trademark of FDN, Inc. © 2007-2016 FDN, Inc. (used with permission).

sense that people think you're a hypochondriac. It feels a bit like maybe they're secretly rolling their eyes, behind your back.

Their words and responses tell you enough. They think you're *kind of pathetic and lazy*. Some of them tell you, "Snap out of it. Pull yourself together."

If only you could. It would be so wonderful. They don't understand how drained you feel. They can't comprehend the guilt you feel over not being able to function. There's simply no reserve of energy left in your body. It's even quite probable your body isn't absorbing nutrients properly.

Most people don't "get" how you have tried everything you can think of, and gone to every doctor you could find who *might* offer help. All to no avail. It's so frustrating. And the worst part? It's how the emotional, physical, and financial aspects gradually mount up and bring you further down. Eventually, depression swallows you.

Emotionally and physically, each day you grow more and more depressed. Your body begins to shut down, piece by piece. Not only can you not function, but your body can no longer repair or heal properly. Your mind becomes so foggy, you can't think straight. A sense of shame envelops you over not being able to take care of the ordinary things.

You gradually see who your real friends are, as many people just disappear out of your life. Apparently, they don't want to "deal with you" anymore. The shame is taxing.

Financially, you'd give anything to recover your life and vitality. You've already invested hundreds, maybe thousands, of dollars in doctors' visits, and still have no answers. It drains your funds, not just your energy. Possibly even worse, many of the doctors won't listen to you. Some of them seem to have a preconceived notion regarding your "case." Others seem to become frustrated with your case, and send you off to some other "specialist," who again, may not listen.

Until a person walks in these shoes of chronic fatigue, (or fibromyalgia, or depression) they will most likely, never fully understand the hellish despair sufferers endure, as they silently wish for answers, which never seem to come. Hope is in short supply.

For me, when my body told me, "*Sleep,*" I had only a minute or so to find a couch or bed, for fear I might pass out cold. When I made it to the couch, I collapsed into deep sleep.

When I woke up, it seemed to be only about an hour later. I was always shocked to realize several hours had slipped by. Other times, I went to bed at night, and slept until 10:00 or 11:00 am. Thinking I'd be OK, I'd go downstairs to start my day, but by the time I got there, the intense fatigue flowed back over me. Suddenly, I needed to sleep again. The couch beckoned.

Hours later I'd awaken and realize it was 3:00 or 4:00 pm. I wondered, "Where did the day go? Jimmy will be coming home from work at any moment."

I was so embarrassed and ashamed. I didn't want him to know all I did was sleep. This pattern continued for about two years.

The Guilt of Not Getting Well

As the sleeping cycle went on, seven days a week, month after month, I kept saying to myself, "I *cannot live* this way."

Jimmy suspected the worst. I wanted to die. I felt living a life on the couch, week in and week out, not being able run the household, or cook and clean for my husband was no life. At this point, I felt like I was a horrible wife, a horrible daughter, a horrible friend, a horrible sister, a horrible human being. I was no good to anyone, not even to myself.

Pain Begets More Pain, Everywhere

As the many months passed, I got worse. I thought by sleeping 15+ hours a day, I would surely get the rest my body needed to replenish and repair. It didn't.

The pain in my body gradually increased. It developed to a point, where I could not even pick up the mop to clean my kitchen floor. I could not take the clothes out of the washing machine and put them in the dryer, without feeling like I had run a marathon.

I thought, *Come on! Really? How sad is this?* Not even the smallest of chores could I perform.

How LOW Could I Go?

Around this time, I finally had to acknowledge, I was indeed, experiencing depression. I had sunk so low, I no longer wanted to deal with any of it. I couldn't say the words out loud, but I wanted to DIE.

WOW! Even as I write this for you, I'm weeping. It's hard to experience the memory of when I felt so awful. I still hate to believe I might have actually acted upon such skewed and stupid thinking.

But I considered it, repeatedly. *How could I do it and not affect anyone? Well, I could make it look like an accident. No one would ever know, right? Would they find me? Would my family be mad?*

What a stupid question. Yes, of course they'd be mad . . . and shocked and disappointed with me. Would they miss me? I am sure they would, but they'd get over it. Would I be better off? Wait . . . Surely God doesn't intend for me to have recently married a wonderful man, and subject him to this. Jimmy doesn't deserve this. This isn't fair to him. God must have a different plan for me, right?

As it turned out, He did have a much better plan for me.

Time for Tough Decisions

Eventually I had to make a tough decision. I could choose death or life. Which one would it be? You can see I chose life. I'm writing about my journey, so you don't have to go through what I did. At least, perhaps I can give you the breadcrumbs to find your way back if you're already there. And there IS a way out from under the black veil depression puts you under, and back into a life worth living.

Next, I spent a lot of time thinking. *How do I pull it all together and figure this out? How do I recover from this downward spiral?*

This was the million-dollar question. Why? Because none of the doctors could figure out what, exactly, was wrong with me. Can you believe it? None of them had a clue how to deal with my decline. I was somehow going to have to solve the dilemma on my own. I would also have to be honest with myself.

The labels doctors came up with, over time, were like a who's who of ailments and disorders. It sometimes seemed as if every time I went to any doctor, they came up with a new "diagnosis" to add to the list. It was crazy.

The very first label, early on, was the urticaria (hives). Then, major depressive disorder, but I was in denial on this one for a very long time. Things went downhill from there.

Then came chronic stress, high blood pressure, and hypothyroidism. The next visits yielded labels of Hashimoto's thyroiditis, obesity, chronic fatigue syndrome, fibromyalgia, and finally they decided I had lupus. But I drew the line there.

I refused to go to the rheumatologist and pay for those tests. It would have meant more drugs and side effects, then more drugs with a few more side effects. At this point, I was done with the guessing game. I was tired of chasing symptoms. It led nowhere but down. I am not a set of labels. I knew there had to be more to it than this.

As I later looked back at things, I found it odd I was willing to accept all the diagnoses, except depression. I had to attempt powering through it. Now I realize the denial was how I tried to avoid the social stigma of depression. Even *I* had a negative concept of it. I didn't want to be seen as "weak" like that. I wanted to been seen more like Wonder Woman.

Depression is something we tend to hear a lot about in the media, and yet no one really wants to talk about it. It's always someone else's unfortunate problem. There is an enormous stigma associated with it. Our society has a crazy view of it. When someone experiences depression, they're supposed to seek help. Yet if they do, the general public tends to look down upon them, like they're weak-minded or feeble. And yet nothing could be further from the truth. It takes incredible courage to seek help navigating out of depression.

What I didn't realize at the time, was how tricky depression is. It tends to cause a skewed sense of self and circumstance. It's a bit like living under a dark veil, so everything in one's life appears darker, and more negative than it really is. It frequently creates an emotional numbness, while also inducing overwhelming sadness. It's a dark place to live.

It not only depresses the mood, demeanor, and experience of the sufferer, but it also depresses the immune system. While I was busy denying my experience of depression, it may well have been contributing to my physical decline. But nobody explained that as a possibility.

To me, it felt as if all the doctors and the psychiatrist were over-emphasizing the depression and treating all the physical suffering like it was in my head. My assortment of symptoms had confounded them. They were stumped. I felt like they were collecting my physical symptoms: fatigue, lack of motivation, emotional numbness, shame, and other general life impairments. Then lumping them into "depression," because they didn't know what else to do with me.

I felt like I wasn't being taken seriously. I suppose, deep down inside, I subconsciously decided denial of the depression was the way to go. That way, they couldn't possibly see me as weak, and they'd have to look more closely at my physical issues. It didn't work so well. I can now see they were trying to take me seriously. They just didn't know how to connect all the symptoms in a way that made sense to them, or to me. They weren't trained to view it all from a holistic perspective.

Meanwhile, the medical bills were mounting up fast, and all for what? None of the labels made any difference. They still couldn't figure out how to "fix" me, and they weren't interested in finding any root causes. The word "frustrated," didn't even come close to describing it.

They continued to fill me with drugs—man-made chemicals— and hoped my body would cooperate with them. They experimented with me, as if I were a guinea pig of little to no value. Month after month, I felt no relief. I kept expecting something to change. I kept hoping and praying something was going to work, and I'd get better. But nothing improved. I wasn't even back at the starting point. I was much worse.

Worse, instead of better? What's wrong with this picture? During my many doctor visits, I'd speak, and no one would listen. All I kept hearing from them was, "OK. Here's a new drug we want you to try. Your bill is $115.00 now, go make your next appointment at the desk, and we'll see you next month."

But what I felt was negated, hushed, and passed over. They just seemed to "pass the buck." None of them appeared interested in what I had to say or how ineffectual their "treatments" were.

It was up to me to figure out how to pull myself up and out of the illness hole. I had more tough decisions—like what to do about the ineffective doctors and their treatments. And how was I going to find help which would actually work for me?

Hey Doc, Please Make Sure Your Ears Are Turned On

I fought the "mainstream practice" as much as I could. I instinctively knew it was not the right path for the amount of healing I needed. Back then, I didn't know what else to do.

I kept expressing, "I want to try something natural. I want to try something without man-made chemicals or drugs in it. Give me something alternative."

Without holistic training, they didn't know how to accommodate me. I didn't know how to find the type of doctor

34

who could work with me in this way. I kept trying to pull them into our working *together*. I only wish they'd been more open to investigating the possibilities. Human "healthcare" is so very odd.

When someone takes their pet to the veterinarian, the first question the vet asks is, "What are you feeding your pet?" It's an extremely valid question. Why don't more people-doctors ask this? What we fuel our body with determines how well it runs. Managing what goes into the body should always be the first step.

Doctors, I plead with you. Please, please listen to, and *hear* your patients. They need wisdom from you. I know you're pressed for time. Perhaps your staff can help you devise better intake questionnaires. Ask your patients probing questions and *really* listen. The clues are there, and you'll discover them when you ask the right questions. Otherwise, you're missing the valuable hints which can guide you both towards a true healing journey. They come to you for healing. This begins with hearing what the patient has to say. Become their health and wellness detective and advocate.

When we, as patients, feel beaten down, and we're barely surviving, it feels like we don't have many choices. As such, we follow what *appears to be* the path of least resistance: the mainstream approach. We don't have the energy we need to play the games, figure out exactly what's required to fight back, or demand answers.

In today's medical landscape, what *looks like* the path of least resistance really isn't. It's backwards, and it's uphill. The true path of least resistance, back to health and wellness, is a holistic track. It's certainly a more balanced approach. However, the more holistic road tends to cost more, because insurance (almost a necessity these days) generally won't play nice with them.

Overall, I did it their way (mainstream medical, allopathic style). I didn't know how to *find* the more holistic practitioners. I wish I'd known then, what I know now.

Chapter 5

A Miracle Unfolds

FROM THE BEGINNING of my adventure, I remember asking God, "Why?" But deep down inside, I knew "why." Somehow, some way, I was going to come back from the "walking-dead." There would be a lesson in all of this—for me, and perhaps for others.

Months before the bottom fell out, I went to my church and was able to see one of the lay pastors for counseling. At the time, I already knew something was wrong with me. But I never imagined my life was about to fall apart. I asked to see someone who wasn't afraid to be truthful with me. I knew I needed to hear the truth, no matter what.

I met with lay Pastor Dick VanCleave. He always gave it to me straight. I am forever grateful for his honesty, compassion and prayers. He's now retired, but I'm glad he gave me God's standard of care. Nothing is impossible for Him.

The Bottom Fell Out

When the bottom fell out of my life, I had multiple doctors. I also had one psychiatrist, and two therapists, at the same time. I was desperate to find out what was wrong with me. By then, I was sleeping almost all day and night. Yet I was always exhausted, no matter how many hours I slept. I could get up, brush my teeth and go right back to bed. Can you imagine becoming so exhausted from just brushing your teeth? Forget doing anything else for yourself.

Overwhelming guilt came over me upon realizing I was neglecting everything. No daily routines. No house cleaning, cooking, or even laundry. I love doing laundry! Yes, I know it's not normal, but I enjoy it.

During the time when I was so sick, I remember if I dropped something on the floor, I didn't have the energy to pick it up. Maybe worse, I really didn't care. This was not me. I am a clean freak, and I love a clean house. Before all this had taken over my life, most days you could practically eat off my floors, if you were so inclined.

What really surprised me the most as my health deteriorated, was how I couldn't verbally communicate. My mind became so befuddled, if you asked me a question, I couldn't form a whole thought, much less express it.

I also remember not *wanting* to talk to anyone—not even my husband, my family, or my friends. It took too much effort. Perhaps because no one really understood what was happening to me. I felt they didn't believe me, or they needed explanations. I didn't have the energy. There was only one person I wanted to try talking to, and that was Pastor Dick.

I don't know why I only cared to communicate with Pastor Dick. I guess deep down inside, I felt he was the only one I could trust. He didn't judge me. He didn't cause me to feel bad, but he would hold me accountable. I wished I could have talked to him every day. Maybe it was because I sensed God's peace in him.

I essentially only spoke if spoken to. Even then, only if it was an easy question. If it took any real brainpower, you could forget about it. I didn't have the clarity to express myself. So I kept quiet. This was not normal for me. Fortunately, as the months progressed, I eventually got my voice back.

The Miracle Surfaces

One day, I woke up from a dead sleep. It was as if angels had whispered in my ear. Out of the blue, I suddenly remembered a movie I had heard of called, *Fat, Sick and Nearly Dead*. I also remembered that we had just recently subscribed to Netflix. I did not even know how to use it yet, but I decided I'd try to figure it out.

Don't ask me how, but somehow I did it. Remember, at this point my thought process was feeling awfully broken. I logged on and searched for the movie. Even though I planned to play the movie, I figured there was no way I would be able to stay awake. Amazingly, when the movie began, something strange happened to me.

Chapter 6

The Catalyst That Ignited the Fire

April 2014—The Documentary That Saved My Life and Changed my Direction:

Fat, Sick and Nearly Dead

JOE CROSS DID the world a humongous favor when he decided to make his documentary, *Fat, Sick and Nearly Dead*.

When the film started, I immediately loved his sense of humor. Starting out with cartoons, he talked about his life. He mentioned he had a condition called urticaria. This instantly sparked my interest. *What? Urticaria? That's Hives! I also have hives.* I was really intrigued. This is a condition you don't generally hear much about.

I was amazed. "Hmmm . . . he *heals* this?"

Years earlier, my dermatologist had basically told me ". . . good luck finding the cause of urticaria." He told me it could flare up at any time. Stress could bring it on, eating could bring it on, and being exposed to the sun would bring it on. Living on Prednisone, a drug I despise, was the only thing that gave me relief. I didn't want to live my life that way.

As Joe's documentary continued, I was practically glued to the television. I actually moved from my normal lying down position to sitting up right. This was a big deal.

Even sitting up, when my body said, "*Sleep!*" I usually started to sleep within a few minutes, but not this time. I was amazingly wide awake. I could not believe what I was seeing. It wasn't what I expected.

This was a documentary about Joe's life, declining health, and finding healing by cutting out the packaged, processed foods and detoxing by only juicing vegetables. I finally realized what I was seeing was my first sign of HOPE in ages. The one thing I had not felt during most of my ordeal.

I watched intently as Joe explained why he chose to detox with juice and document his experience. I cried through most of the movie. Not because it's sad. But because for the first time in months, I was seeing an answer to my prayers, feeling hope, and visualizing a potential action plan.

This was a possible way out of my horrible ordeal. Juicing vegetables for six months was not an easy way to live, but if it worked, then I didn't care what I had to do.

"I will do it!"

As the piece ended, I turned on my computer and I looked up Joe Cross. I saw he was hosting a juicing boot camp in New York the next month. I called my mom and told her about it. She's always up for healthy living and loves to juice. She told me she couldn't go, because she was taking care of my great aunt.

When Jimmy came home, I told him about the documentary and the boot camp. He told me if I wanted to go, then I should. I thought about it and figured, what else was I doing but sleeping all day long? It wasn't like I had to make room in my schedule.

As exciting as it was, I was also scared. At the time, I couldn't go even an hour without sleeping. I could barely take care of myself, or think clearly. Yet I was considering flying to New York and attending a juicing boot camp.

I thought, *There's No way. But I've got to try.*

I made a few phone calls and said to myself, *I am so desperate to get my life back. I have to take the chance and do this.*

I booked the room and the flight. I was scared beyond belief to be traveling by myself. Even though it was something I've done alone for years and had no problem, now things were so different. I was set to attend the next boot camp, in May 2014.

Prep Work

I learned before you can attend this boot camp, you must start to eliminate foods in your diet, to begin the detox process. I had signed up so late, my initial detox window was very small. I didn't care. I assembled the list and started to prep immediately.

There were two reasons I didn't care about my short detox window: 1) I didn't want travel so far and have to detox while there. 2) I felt the odds were already against me. I wasn't even functioning in my day-by-day life, but could I fly so many miles and detox simultaneously? I was afraid they would have to admit me to a hospital.

I wasn't driving by then, so Jimmy took me to the grocery store with my prep list. It was nothing but vegetables. I shopped and started outlining my prep. I believe hope brought the excitement I needed to start my progress back to health. Hope is a powerful thing. A grocery list or eating plan was something I'd never received from any of my doctors, much less any shreds of hope.

I don't remember how much my grocery bill was that day. I didn't care, as long as it would help me. Even though I felt a little bad that Jimmy had to drive me everywhere and do so much for me, I was grateful. Miss Independent was on sabbatical, but that's just how it was for the time.

I started my detox the next day. Vegetable, after vegetable, after vegetable. It wasn't as bad as you might think. Actually, I was enjoying some really good food. Who would have thought?

Departure time approached. I packed and prepped, and I went off for the adventure of my life—Juicing Boot Camp. It was so scary. I didn't know a soul there, and would be rooming with a stranger. Additionally, I was still in my mummy sleeping stage. I couldn't go but a few minutes at a time without falling asleep when my body demanded it. I didn't care. I was determined to do this, somehow, no matter what.

Chapter 7

Boot Camp, Here I Come

Rebooting Myself, at Boot Camp

I KNEW THERE would be people from all over the world going to this juicing boot camp. I arrived at the airport in New York and saw them assembling near the shuttle terminal. The shuttle would take us to the Omega Institute in Rhinebeck, NY, where the boot camp was being held.

I noticed all the participants arrived in pretty much the same shape. We were sick, and dealing with various ailments. I met some really nice people and made a friend to hang out with. Once we arrived at the Omega Institute, we walked around campus. It was so beautiful—the fresh air, the mountains, the entire campus—it was gorgeous and peaceful. We scoped it out and learned our way around.

We had free time and one last meal before the juicing began. We found the dining hall for our "Last Supper." From that point forward, we would only eat boot-camp-friendly meals. They were listed on the bar, so we knew what we could have. It was the best food I'd ever tasted. Trust me. I'm a foodie, and I'm picky.

I wondered why this food was so good. I couldn't understand, but I was about to find out.

"Boot camp friendly" meant vegetarian—vegetables on top of more vegetables. I don't think I even saw pasta. I don't remember vegetables ever being this delicious before. The food was so good that I was determined to find the chef and discover his secret. I did manage to get a few recipes. I wanted to be able to duplicate some of those wonderful choices, once I returned home.

Let the Juicing Begin!

The next morning, I learned we'd start with a glass of warm water infused with ginger and lemon. We lined up with our provided juice cups, and received our prepared juice. Behind the scenes, several people were juicing thousands of pounds of carrots, ginger, sweet potatoes, oranges, spinach, cucumber, and all manner of other vegetables. Once we picked up our juice, we proceeded to the lecture hall where the meetings were to take place. The speakers were the next best thing about juicing camp.

My new friend, Lori, and I walked into the large lecture hall and decided where we would sit.

"Hey Lori, we've paid a lot of money to be here. I'm too sick to miss any of this. I want to sit up front, so we can get the most from it."

She agreed. We were front and center for all the lectures presented that week.

The Phrase That Changed My Thinking

I had no idea when I arrived at boot camp, it would completely change the direction of my life. I learned an entirely new way of thinking. Each day we had different speakers give lectures on various topics. They taught us new food theories—eating vegan, vegetarian, and raw foods, as well as nutrition for thyroid support, just to name a few.

I also learned surprising things regarding food science, and the psychology of food. They gave us tremendous amounts of information to take home. So many enlightening theories were outlined, some I'd never heard of.

One thing which really resonated within me, down through my deepest core, was a quote by Hippocrates, "Let food be thy medicine, and medicine be thy food."

When I saw the quote, it intrigued me. Using food as medicine? What an amazing idea! I could do this and not have to use prescriptions? Wow.

Remember, I had said from the beginning, I wanted to find the root causes as well as use a natural way to heal my body. Here it was. The one thing doctors *never* talked to me about was *nutrition*. And yet, one thing we do, every day, usually three times a day, *We EAT.*

I couldn't stop thinking about this. *Food as medicine.* My wheels were really turning.

Why had no one else thought to bring this to my attention before? I'd never really heard this, or if I had, it never resonated within me.

Where My Journey Took Off and the Light Went On

On about the third day at camp, something happened for me. The only way I can really explain it is to say that while I was sick, I knew deep down inside there was something terribly wrong with me. I just couldn't put my finger on it. By the third day, something switched on, in my brain. I never realized it was turned off, until I felt the difference. I can't explain the feeling. I only know I felt a shift take place.

We had been placed into groups with similar health conditions. Everyone in my group said they could see the difference in me. It was like my internal light bulb had not been fully powered. Then suddenly, the power was restored to my physical and mental processes, and it shined brightly. My group members told me they could see the light come on in my eyes.

Yet another big surprise at camp was I did not need to sleep all day. I wondered how that was possible. How did the need for so much sleep just go away? How did I suddenly have energy for the first time in several months? Additionally, I didn't feel like crying all day, and my mind felt so much clearer. I could actually process my thoughts. I felt so much better.

There had to be some truth to, "Let food be thy medicine, and medicine be thy food."

All the juicing, eating a vegetarian diet, and eliminating processed foods, seemed to increase my energy dramatically. The "light bulb" kept getting brighter in my mind. Food can either cause disease, or heal disease.

Wow! This stuff really needed further study.

As the week went on, I was waking up at 6 am. Long ago, this had been normal for me—not my recent sleeping until 10 or 11 am, or going right back to bed.

If I could keep this up for the rest of my life, I'd be so happy.

I was actually *talking* to people and sharing. I loved the experience so much. I thought if I could go to this boot camp every year, I'd love it. I would recommend it to everyone.

The Food Detective is On the Job

My new food inquisition continued. By then, my detective mind was engaging. I was asking questions like a 2-year old kid, wanting to know why this, and why that. Let's start with the juicing.

When I experienced juicing at boot camp, I realized I'd been missing something while doing it at home. What was so different from my home juicing? I soon found the answer.

Organic vegetables and fruits make a HUGE difference. You might wonder, as I had, is there really a difference using locally grown and harvested? And yes, there is.

The lectures answered all of my questions. I learned how to buy organic fruits and vegetables on a budget. I learned about *the dirty dozen*—conventionally grown vegetables and fruits that contain the highest amounts of pesticides and chemical fertilizers.

And I learned about *the clean 15*—vegetables and fruits that tend to be safer from the pesticides. They generally have thicker skins, or the parts we eat are not directly exposed to the chemicals. They usually have a lower pesticide and chemical load. Therefore, we should be budgeting to buy organic for *the dirty dozen,* but we can be lax about buying organic with *the clean 15,* as they are already a bit safer.

I learned about C.S.A. groups—community supported agriculture. This is where I learned a lot more regarding ways to save money on produce. There was *so* much education in such a short time. I learned the science behind organic nutrition, and I better understood why we should eat organic foods. Even with all this education, I still could not get enough. I became a sponge. The juicing camp ended up giving me all the solid foundation I needed going forward.

While I was enjoying myself at camp, I also learned about a nutrition school, The Institute for Integrative Nutrition®. Of all things, a school for holistic nutrition. I had no idea such a thing existed. At that point, I didn't realize the direction my life was about to take. I didn't see the tremendous changes taking place, nor the upcoming changes that were saving my life.

When I left Juicing Boot Camp 2014, I was so excited to feel *normal* for the first time in years.

Normal? What is normal? Wait! My old normal was sleeping, feeling exhausted, and not being able to move. This new normal was fantastic.

I felt like I did in my 20's. I was happy, feeling great, having energy, and not needing to sleep all day. I found myself giving the kitchen a good, thorough cleaning, for the first time in many months. I was singing and dancing to Latin music.

Unfortunately, this changed within a few weeks of returning home. I didn't realize how tough it would be to maintain my great, positive, new habits once back in "the real world." When I experienced being back with family and friends, it turned out to be hard to stay on track.

Everyone else had been doing the same ol' stuff, and eating the same ol' processed junk. Before long, processed food sneaked back into my diet, as did a few other things I *knew* I should stay away from. But it was difficult to be around so many of the "bad" foods I used to enjoy.

What I did next, finalized the process of my journey back to health.

Chapter 8

Institute for Integrative Nutrition® Saves Lives

Bottomed Out, Again?

I WAS MAD at myself. Within a few weeks of being home from my wonderful experience at boot camp, my good habits deteriorated, and I bottomed out again. It was another downward spiral, back into lacking energy, and needing to sleep more and more. But this time, because I'd learned so much at boot camp, I was able to recognize I needed to get back on track in a sustainable way. I realized I had to find my next step.

I had now truly grasped what a positive difference whole food makes. The next step changed my life forever. It taught me the sustainability I needed to stay on track.

Learning About the Institute for Integrative Nutrition® (IIN®)

Before I tell you about this next step, I want to share something with you. If it were not for learning about the Institute for Integrative Nutrition®, I would not be here now. IIN® is not only amazing, it's a life changer. I am forever grateful for learning about it at boot camp, and for all I learned at IIN®. I'm so thankful for the various theories and strategies to which I was exposed, and that I was able to apply to my life. This school covers it all, and then some.

The Push to Go All In

I decided the next step had to be finding that nutrition school. I went online to look up the Institute for Integrative Nutrition® website: Here is my direct link: http://geti.in/1zbWHbz

Once I was at the website, I felt another glimmer of hope. I got excited again and called my mom. She has always been my biggest cheerleader and promoter of health. She's the one who always supports me and who has no problem telling me when I'm wrong, even when I don't want to hear it.

I told her about this school I'd found that teaches nutrition in a different way. I told her I was considering attending. Once again, I didn't know how I would be able to do it, because of all the sleep my body required. But I figured if I had managed getting through Joe's Juicing Boot Camp, I could do this from home. I didn't have to go anywhere. In between hours of sleep, I could focus my best attempt at the class work. When I needed to sleep, I would.

I told my mom, I felt I had a choice. I could either spend the last few dollars I had on doctors, who had not helped me so far, or I could invest in myself. When I phrased it like that, how could I not invest in myself?

Since leaving my job in early 2013, I had no income. Thank God I had saved some money for a rainy day. But I knew I would still need financial help. I asked my mom for some assistance.

My mom hated seeing what I'd been through, and how the life had been sucked out of me. She could tell I wasn't the same vibrant, sassy, outgoing, overachiever she had raised. She was onboard with my decision. She told me she would contribute and I was so grateful to have her support. The next person I approached was not initially as supportive as I hoped.

The next day, I decided to discuss it with my Jimmy. I told him about the online nutrition and health coaching school. His reaction was . . . well . . . just about as I expected, but not what I'd hoped for. It wasn't that he didn't support me, he was simply resistant. He told me he didn't want me to do it, and I could see the concern in his expression. He knew how lousy and tired I'd been feeling, and I think he was worried I'd take on too much, and the stress would cause me to get worse.

He could see what had happened to me. I had deteriorated into this sick person he'd been living with for months. He could see I wasn't the same sparkly person he had known for years before. He watched me take a chance traveling to boot camp and feeling so much better, only to deteriorate again. I'm sure it was scary for him to watch. All I could tell him was how desperately I wanted to regain the good health I'd had upon returning home from boot camp. I must to try this.

While I appreciated his concern, he didn't fully understand the anguish burning deep within my soul—the desperation to become whole again. I wanted so much more for my life. I had been a wife who took care of her home and husband, and handled everyday responsibilities. I yearned to do that again, but I was too sick now. It was like my internal flame was suffocating, and I had to find a way to revive it and bring it back to it's healthy, brilliant state again.

The determination inside me, to be whole again, made it that much more desirable to do this nutrition school thing. After my discussion with Jimmy, I decided to do what any other formerly-sassy, sick, desperate, person would do. Give up? No, not exactly.

I woke up the next morning, made the phone call to the IIN®, and signed up. My class started in July 2014.

Jimmy always laughs at me. He tells me if he wanted to buy a new boat or motorcycle, and I told him, "No," he wouldn't get them. I, on the other hand, wouldn't listen if he told me, "No." He knows he would come home and find them in the garage.

But I felt strongly about the IIN® health coaching school, and it was nothing like a boat or a motorcycle. This was my life I was trying to reclaim. I needed help figuring out how I could sustainably implement the Hippocrates quote: "Let food be thy medicine, and medicine be thy food." I was realizing I had to take responsibility for healing myself. Only I could do this.

I imagine plenty of people can go home from boot camp and pull off the dietary changes in their life. But I'd had trouble integrating those changes, once I was home. I felt strongly that I could learn even more valuable information from this school. It was the next logical step for me to continue learning what I'd started at boot camp. That's probably why they told us about it.

I was tired of getting no healing from the western medical community. I had to figure this out, and I had a feeling attending IIN® was going to help me put it all together. Besides, I could be my first client.

Back to School

I was so excited for the learning experience ahead of me. I was hungry for as much knowledge as I could retain. Every week, our new modules and lectures opened up for our access. I couldn't wait to learn more than 100 different dietary theories. I was eager to learn from the likes of forward-thinking people like Dr. Mark Hyman, Dr. Mehmet Oz, Dr. Andrew Weil, and Deepak Chopra MD. These experts were among so many others in this growing field of Integrative and Functional Health.

Each week my mind opened to new theories. I decided I would try them all. And I did. Even if it was only one meal, I planned to try as many as I could. I ate vegetarian. I ate vegan. I ate meat. I tried the Blood Type Diet. I ate local. I ate raw food. I tried just about everything.

I was my own lab rat, and I was going to learn, once and for all, what worked for my body, and what didn't. Jimmy had to come along with me on this journey, like it or not. Thank God he loves food. He had no problem eating what I put in front of him. He started enjoying some of the new foods I made.

I learned no one is exactly the same as another. One person's food could be another person's poison. We are all biochemically just a little different. This is why what may be good for me, might not be the best food for someone else. IIN® left no stone unturned. They covered it all.

Sometimes, it was difficult to decipher which dietary theory was best for me. I had to experiment to discover what my body liked. Only I could translate which foods gave me energy, and which made me sluggish and tired.

One of the best lectures I remember was from David Wolfe. He is what I call the guru of raw food. When he gave his lecture, the light bulbs in my head started to fire up again. That's when I realized the chaos going on inside my body was a bigger deal than I'd suspected. I needed to heal it as quickly as possible.

David Wolfe teaches about eating 'superfoods' and raw food. Yes, raw vegetables and fruits, along with healthy fats. The thing I liked about his lecture was how he showed us what he was talking about. I could see what he was doing, and it made sense. He wasn't just talking, he was teaching about juicing and blending. He stressed the benefits of superfoods in our diets, and how easy it could be to add them.

I watched intently as he took a coconut, cut it open, and put the meat and juice in the Vitamix®—a really good, emulsifying blender. He added various superfoods, talked about the benefits, and why we should all eat raw foods. I loved that he taught us how to do this properly, because most of us growing up in the US wouldn't know the procedure. I was a bit more familiar with coconuts, because I often visited Puerto Rico as a child. But his lecture clarified the process greatly.

I thought about what I was seeing and decided, why not try this as well? I couldn't honestly say I wouldn't like it until I tried it.

I went to Whole Foods Market and bought a coconut. I cut it just like he showed us in his lecture and put it in my Vitamix®. I added superfoods, blended it all together, and drank it.

I was amazed. After I drank the superfood smoothie, something wild happened to me. For the first time in 3 months, I had energy, and I wasn't hungry for hours. That's when I put it together. I was gradually discovering the root of my problem. I had learned the nutrients in the food I was eating were not being properly absorbed.

I realized then, I was dealing with something called 'leaky gut.' I'd heard of it many times, also referred to as intestinal permeability. It was not until that moment that it really sank into my brain—I was dealing with leaky gut. OMG!

What is leaky gut? One source describes it like this:

"Leaky gut syndrome (LGS) or intestinal permeability syndrome (IPS) is a gastro intestinal dysfunction caused by increased permeability of the intestinal wall, which allows absorption of toxic material–bacteria, fungi, parasites, etc. LGS may be linked to allergy and various autoimmune conditions."[8]

What? Allow me to explain it in layman's terms.

For a moment, think of your intestines like a house with brick walls. Ideally, the brick walls keep out the light, wind, rain, dust, bugs, raccoons, uninvited people, and other unpleasant potential invaders. They also keep out the heat of summer or the cold of winter. The intact walls protect you from the outside world.

If your brick walls develop holes in the mortar, between the joints of brick, suddenly those outside elements—the light, wind, rain, dust, and bugs—can get through. If bigger holes develop, then larger bugs, lizards, and other small wildlife could get in. The more gaps in a wall, the more unwanted things get into your house. Now you're no longer protected from the outside world.

This is a very basic analogy of what is going on inside your intestines. As the food you eat travels through your digestive system, it is gradually broken down for your intestines to absorb nutrients. But when you develop gaps in the wall of your

---

[8] Segen's Medical Dictionary. S.v. "Leaky gut." Retrieved April 2, 2016 from http://medical-dictionary.thefreedictionary.com/Leaky+gut

intestines, a couple of things happen. One, not as many nutrients can be absorbed, causing undernourishment, even though you may be eating a healthy diet. Two, lots of things pass through those gaps, and into your body which are never supposed to be there—causing inflammation.

Things that get through those gaps are food particles, bacteria, fungi, and viruses, to name a few. Once they get though the gaps, they are floating around in your body. The immune system then tries to deal with them as foreign invaders. This is how your body develops food sensitivities, food allergies, and some inflammation.

A new world of understanding opened up for me when I realized I was probably dealing with leaky gut. It dawned on me this problem was only the beginning—the tip of the proverbial iceberg. What I was about to learn in the next few months changed my view of food.

Through my IIN® modules, I continued learning about all manner of food allergies and sensitivities, some of which I had developed over the years. Turns out, stress plays a role in that as well. I'd been clueless about it, until I understood the mechanics behind it. Then it began to make sense. By this point, I had to start eliminating certain foods, in order to heal my gut.

I'm a foodie, and I love good quality, great tasting food. So I thought this elimination thing would be awful. It sounds worse than it really is. It required me to change my entire diet. I learned about swaps and replacements. I gave up processed food (no food out of a can or a box). I ate only whole foods. I learned to enjoy food like I'd never known before. I was trying new things and loving it. After a couple of days, I didn't miss processed food anymore.

As I continued my modules from week to week, each lecture taught me to add new things in my diet. I learned to remove things, and I learned to cook in new ways. I learned to live life with a new foundation of knowledge. I tried every dietary theory, whether it made sense to me or not. I needed to know what would work for my body.

After three months at IIN®, I was able to wean down from sleeping 15+ hours a day. I went from lying down and listening to my lectures, to sitting up straight. Then I went from sitting up to walking a few minutes at a time. By mid-October 2014, I had progressed to listening to my lectures on the treadmill.

As I write this for you, I can now walk five miles a day, clean my house, go grocery shopping, spend time with my husband— all in one day, and *not* have to sleep several times. I wish I could share more about what I learned at IIN®, but it would be a volume in and of itself, too large to read here.

All I can say is, "Thank you Joshua Rosenthal, for coming up with this school and showing me how to get my life back."

As I completed those first three months of IIN®, my husband began to see differences. He wondered if this was for real, and what was going on with me. I dare not say more than that. If you want to hear what happened, you'll have to invite me to come speak to your group. It's a doozy of a story. Only a few people have heard it. It's funny, but it's personal.

During the next three months, more changes occurred. By January 2015, I was able to move around the house with less pain. That's when I decided it was time to really get moving. I had already started walking, but this is when I worked it up to walking five miles at a time.

I was loving it. The next three months, I saw even more changes. By April 2015, I found I actually wanted to talk to people. I know that sounds so simple, but remember at one point, I couldn't really speak, think, or express what was in my head. I had pulled inside myself, like a turtle. This was a big turnaround for me. The depression was disappearing, little by little. I was getting my life back, in short bursts. I started making friends again. Things were looking better and better.

I still worked on my diet. I tweaked it, week by week. By then, I realized I had some food allergies. I learned to listen to my body and eliminate the foods which were not good for me. I finally gave up gluten. After two days without gluten in my diet, I felt normal for the first time in a long time.

I never realized I was allergic or sensitive to gluten. I've learned that's pretty common. Later I found out why. Growing up eating the Standard American Diet (SAD), amounted to numerous poor dietary choices over the years. In this way, I had somehow turned on one of the celiac genes in my body.

I continued gradually eliminating foods that I suspected were problematic, but I never put it all together—until IIN® taught me about food sensitivities, and listening to my body.

Months later I finally began seeing the biggest difference in my life. I was losing weight, and feeling better. I decided with all the education in nutrition, it was time to explore what was going on inside my body.

I'd learned about the digestion process through IIN®, and it piqued my interest. I wanted to learn more, so I read more. As I mentioned earlier, I was fairly certain I was dealing with leaky gut. Now that I understood more about digestion, I wanted to find out if leaky gut was actually an issue for me.

This happened at the same time my long-time friend, Leah, crossed my path again. She had access to special testing. Through that we learned I was, indeed, dealing with leaky gut, along with several food sensitivities. All the recent stressors I'd lived through had disrupted my digestive process to the point it was no longer working properly. Additionally, my nutrients were not being absorbed correctly.

As my year at IIN® concluded in July 2015, my life was getting back on track. I was excited and no longer just a spectator in my own life. As I made further changes along the way, everything in my world improved.

Chapter 9

My Circle of Life

One of the best assignments, which showed my progress throughout my year at IIN®, was a tool they call "The Circle of Life[9]." It was developed by IIN®. I'll show it to you on the following pages.

It measures twelve areas of satisfaction levels in your life. It also introduces a concept they call the "Primary Foods" and the "Secondary Foods," which I'll explain shortly.

I now use these tools in my Integrative Nutrition® Health Coaching practice. It helps my clients see, and appreciate their surprising progress along the way.

It's been said that you cannot change what you don't measure. I believe The Circle of Life is a prime example of one of the perfect measuring tools.

By measuring the progress over three, six, nine, and twelve months, you can see for yourself all the good you've done. This is why I find it to be such a valuable tool, and why I use it with my clients. Let me show you.

---

[9] The Circle of Life, Primary Food(s), and Secondary Food(s): © 2005 Integrative Nutrition, Inc. (used with permission).

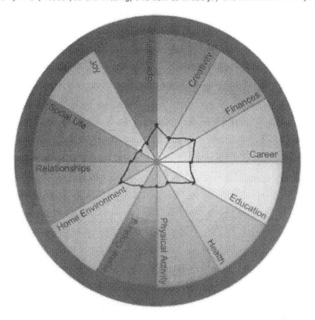

THE CIRCLE OF LIFE *One month (Starting Point)*

Discover which primary foods you are missing, and how to infuse joy and satisfaction into your life.

Figure 1: My 1st Circle of Life during, 1st month of classes.

The way this tool works is to examine how you feel about each area (depicted) of your life. The more satisfied you are in an indicated area, the closer to the outside edge the point should be. Conversely, the least satisfied you are, the closer to the center the points will fall in each area. Then, you simply connect the dots.

Here above, is my beginning Circle of Life[10] exercise. I did this in my first month at IIN®. Since the points were all near the center of the circle at that time, it indicated there was a great deal of dissatisfaction in the various areas of my life. You can see, I was a bit of a mess.

---

[10] The Circle of Life: © 2005 Integrative Nutrition, Inc. (used with permission).

THE CIRCLE OF LIFE

Discover which primary foods you are missing, and how to infuse joy and satisfaction into your life.

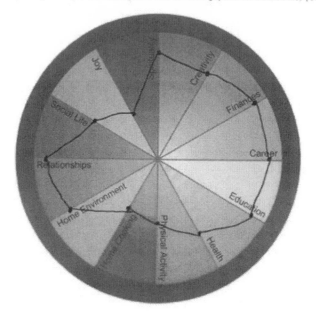

Figure 2: My 3-month Circle of Life assignment.

Above is my 3-month Circle of Life[11] exercise. You can already see quite the difference as the points were gradually migrating outward—to healthier spots, near the outside edge of The Circle.

I wish you could see it in color. But if you decide you'd like to learn more about it, I do use these with my clients. Feel free to contact me.

---

[11] The Circle of Life: © 2005 Integrative Nutrition, Inc. (used with permission)

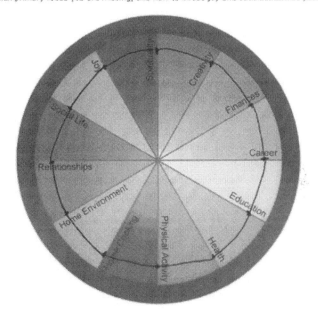

THE CIRCLE OF LIFE

Discover which primary foods you are missing, and how to infuse joy and satisfaction into your life.

Figure 3: My 6-month Circle of Life assignment.

And here, you can see even more progress in my Circle of Life[12] at the 6-month mark. Interestingly, the more I learned about heathy options, and the best lifestyle changes for me to make, the more I evened-out my satisfaction in the various areas of life that we were measuring.

---

[12] The Circle of Life: © 2005 Integrative Nutrition, Inc. (used with permission).

THE CIRCLE OF LIFE

Discover which primary foods you are missing, and how to infuse joy and satisfaction into your life.

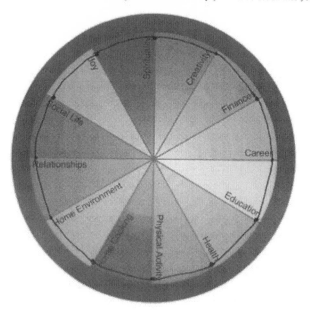

Figure 4: My final Circle of Life assignment at 9-months.

As you can see from my last Circle of Life[13] above, at the 9-month mark, there was a dramatic difference from where I'd begun. I could hardly believe how far I'd come.

Some people might make faster or slower progress, depending on what things they decide need the most focus at any given time. It's certainly possible to use more than four measuring periods within a year. You could even measure your progress each month, if you decided it would be more helpful. Everyone is a bit different.

---

[13] The Circle of Life: © 2005 Integrative Nutrition, Inc. (used with permission).

Over the months, as you make various changes and adjustments in your life, it can feel like a regular day-to-day thing. It may not seem like you're doing much that would make enough of a difference. But as you measure what you're doing, you can see how far you've come and where further adjustments might need to be made.

During each module, I was learning so many great things at IIN®. It could have been overwhelming, but it wasn't. Each month I added a few more of the new ideas I'd learned. This tool brought it all together.

In the beginning, I might not have known where to start. But early on, once they taught us about The Circle of Life[14], I could see and measure my areas of imbalance. Then I knew where to focus my implementation of my positive changes, for the best results. As I made the adjustments I could see my progress.

Now I'll explain more about the twelve categories that The Circle of Life measures, and how we learned to adjust them.

---

[14] The Circle of Life: © 2005 Integrative Nutrition, Inc. (used with permission).

(Chapter 9.5)
The Circle of Life,
Primary Foods, and Secondary Foods[15]

Here is a blank view of the Circle of Life[16]. Notice the twelve life categories this tool measures. I'll list them for you.

The twelve categories in the Circle of Life are: creativity, finance, career, education, health, physical activity, home cooking, home environment, relationships, social life, joy, and spirituality. Out these twelve, the four *main* ones are: career, relationships, physical activity, and spirituality.

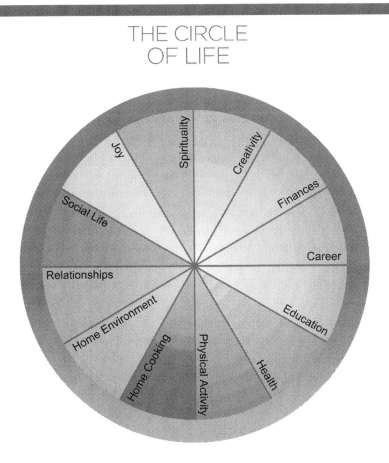

© INTEGRATIVE NUTRITION

---

[16] The Circle of Life: © 2005 Integrative Nutrition, Inc. (used with permission).

As I promised, here are the explanations of the concepts of Primary Foods and Secondary Foods[17]. It might surprise you a little.

According to IIN®, Primary Foods are—surprisingly—not even food at all.

Sometimes when we think we're hungry for food, we're actually hungry for something else. Our mind, body, and emotions are looking for sustenance and balance.

Whereas Secondary Foods are the nutrients we ingest—the food we eat.

I actually tried this theory out. I spent the entire day with a very good friend of mine, my college roommate Monika. At the end of the day we both noticed we had not eaten much, and we weren't even hungry. That's when we realized what we needed— rather than food—was the nourishment our mutual friendship provided.

Quality time spent with a loved one (a healthy relationship) is a Primary Food source. This is where the Circle of Life comes in handy. Fill yours out and see what could be lacking in your life. Could it be that your spiritual life needs attention? Are you happy with your work situation? Do you get enough exercise daily? Are you in a healthy relationship? If not, start making small changes and dig deeper.

I was not aware that my Primary Foods were out of order. Once I knew, I started making small changes. Within months, my happiness grew beyond belief. When you figure this out, then you can look at your Secondary Foods[18].

---

[17] The Circle of Life, Primary Food(s), and Secondary Food(s): ©2005 Integrative Nutrition, Inc. (used with permission).

[18] Primary Food(s) and Secondary Food(s): ©2005 Integrative Nutrition, Inc. (used with permission).

Now when you are hungry, think about it. Are you actually hungry for food, or is your Primary Food out of order?

If you have questions about Primary or Secondary Foods, write them down and send me a note. I'd be happy to explore this with you. It's fascinating, once you start looking deeper at it.

Chapter 10

'Dr. No Hope'

OK, STICK WITH me here, because we have to go back a little bit in the chronology of my story. It's somewhere in the middle of 2012—I've started seeing various doctors, including a new primary care physician along with my therapist, Pastor Dick.

After a year with this new primary care doc, the things she had prescribed weren't working. She decided it was time for me to seek out someone with more expertise in prescribing higher doses of antidepressants.

I expressed my preference to see a Christian practitioner. She didn't have anyone who fit that description. In speaking with Pastor Dick about my dilemma, he gave me a few recommendations. When I told my primary doc about my pastor's list of possibilities, she agreed that was the next best step.

Early 2013 was the last time I saw her.

I chose one of the recommendations, and I set the appointment to see the psychiatrist. I know this may seem counterintuitive to you, as you read this now. You might be asking yourself, "Well if she wanted to go an alternative route, then why did she agree to see someone who might be prescribing higher dosages of pharmaceuticals?"

I get your confusion. But please understand—I was feeling incredibly broken. I had so much trouble thinking and speaking up. What little voice I had left, was so weak, no one would listen. I was so insanely fatigued that I had virtually no energy, and certainly not enough energy for going to battle for myself. So I acquiesced, and went were they nudged me to go.

When my husband took me to see the psychiatrist in spring of 2013, I already had Pastor Dick on my health team. But this new psychiatrist assigned another therapist to me. She worked in his building, across the hall. I did as I was told—too tired to argue. Fortunately, I happened to like her.

In my own mind, I called this psychiatrist 'Dr. No Hope' (not his real name, of course). I told him I didn't want to take prescription medication, that I wanted to find the root cause of my condition. I asked him to find an alternative to using antidepressants—maybe supplements.

He was uncomfortable with 'alternative' approaches. He didn't think they worked. He had no experience in natural treatments. He had studied the usual, allopathic approach of the vast majority of doctors. Since he'd attended school years ago, integrative medical approaches were too new for him. He didn't know what the alternatives really were.

Every visit, I had the same discussion with him. I wanted to find the root cause(s), and he wanted to medicate symptoms. Each visit, he played a guessing game and gave me a new medication that didn't work. Every time, I felt no one was listening to me.

I felt hopeless and ashamed—and very frustrated. I wanted to scream at him, *"Listen* to what I am trying to tell you." But he never really got it. At this time, I was still unable to adequately express myself, and my thinking was still scrambled. I could hear my thoughts, but the words would not come out of my mouth. Believe me, I tried.

Finally, my husband stopped driving me because he had to work. I didn't want him to take any more time off. It was hard for me to drive, but I did it. I went in and cried, due to the frustration of not being able to say what was on my mind in the way I wanted to say it.

I needed to find the right answers, because something inside me was desperate to heal. I never wanted to go through this again. Fearing this state of illness might never end, I kept on saying the same thing, "I want the root cause. I want the root cause." I didn't know how else to express it. My psychiatrist didn't know how to address it.

Deep inside I must have known this was more than a simple psychiatric issue. I felt there were physical components that labeling it as "depression" didn't begin to address. Somehow, I knew there were significant problems in my body that were being ignored by the psychiatrist. All he could see was the depression. He couldn't see the whole body-mind component. He was never trained to see that kind of connection.

The stress of driving myself was bad enough, but to not have Jimmy's support during my visits was another stressor. I remember one of my first few visits without him. As usual, I wanted to learn of alternative ways to heal my condition. My psychiatrist decided to tell me what he considered the alternatives to be.

We discussed shock treatment. Really? In this day and age? But I now realize there has been a great deal of advancement in this area.

I remember listening to him as he told me this treatment could induce seizures. I will never forget that visit. It was the day I thought I would commit suicide after I left.

Yes, I wanted to kill myself. If all I had to look forward to was shock treatments and seizures, then why not? I went home and thought of different ways I could leave this life behind. Then I remembered my relationship with God. I realized this was not God's plan for my life.

Knowing I was in for the fight of my life, I finally told myself, "The time to figure this out is now."

I continued to see the psychiatrist for many months, disappointed and frustrated every session. I never felt any better, only worse. Hope was in short supply. All he seemed to know how to do was toss random, toxic chemicals at my symptoms.

At one point, about half-way through my time with this psychiatrist, I brought a book to him. I wanted him to read *The UltraMind Solution*, by Dr. Mark Hyman, MD. My understanding was that he liked and respected Dr. Mark Hyman. I thought it would be a good way for my psychiatrist to understand what kind of approach I'd been asking for, and that it had a sound medical premise. I'm pretty sure he flipped through it a few times, but I don't know that he ever read the book—at least not while I was his patient.

During the same timeframe, I saw the therapist the doc had assigned to me. She shared his office space, and I liked her. She actually listened to me. She also prayed with me every visit. She was open-minded and willing to talk about real alternative treatments. She told me to talk to the doctor, regarding the other options she and I discussed. But my psychiatrist was not open to them.

After many months, my psychiatrist finally caved and ordered one of the alternative tests my therapist had suggested. I was given the paperwork for a test my insurance company would not reimburse. As it turns out, most of the alternative lab tests are not covered by insurance. I could see the expression on his face. He did not have faith in the tests and believed there would be no success using them. It was disheartening to see his lack of faith in this science.

Visit after visit, I watched the process we fell into, as if I were a spectator. I asked questions, and my psychiatrist answered me with nonsense. (At the time it felt more like . . . well . . . I'll be polite and not spell out BS). I didn't like his thinking, and I started challenging it, as best I could. I learned to read him, instead of him reading me.

I could actually see when he lied to me as he answered many of my questions. He told me what he wanted me to believe. I think he was trying to banish the alternative treatment stuff from my head. I never said anything to anyone about it. I started praying and asking God for help.

And just a few weeks later, He answered me. It was a 'chance' encounter. I happened to be visiting my mom, in Florida.

When I lived there, I was close to a very lovely lady named Leah, but I hadn't seen her in years. That day, I was on my way to pick up my mom. Something caused me to make an unscheduled stop—there was Leah—and everything changed.

Chapter 11

More Miracles: Leah

As I PROGRESSED through this journey, my eyes were opened a little more each day. I learned to look for the miracles in my life. When all this started, I could not see the hand of God in my life. It's not because He wasn't there, it's because I was too sick to see it. I was unable to decipher the signs, and see Him working in the background. I believe this was because God was carrying me.

Re-Aligning Me with a Much-Needed Resource

Once my life began changing and my health was gradually improving a little (thanks to my dietary improvements), I decided to visit my mother in Florida for a few days. She had moved there from New York, a couple of years after my dad passed away.

One day, Mom needed to babysit my two nephews, so I borrowed her car. I decided I would stop at the mall for some lunch. It was about 45 minutes from my mom's house, but still on the way. When I arrived at the mall, I chose Nordstrom's for some of my favorite soup. It was a special place for me because back when I was living in Florida, I used to meet a dear friend at this place. It brought back fond memories.

I ordered my soup and turned around to look for a table. When I turned around, there was my *miracle*. My dear friend Leah, and her daughter Hayley, sat at a table right in front of me. They were there having lunch as well, even though this place was about 45 minutes in the opposite direction from where they lived.

Perhaps most people would consider this to be a chance encounter. But I knew it was a Divine appointment for both of us.

Leah and I go way back to before she had children. I was about 18 or 19 years old when I met her. We've kept in touch over these past 25-30 years. I remember each of her children—playing with them, chasing them around the house, and yes, changing their diapers too. Now grown, it was nice to see them in a different phase of life.

I was so happy to see Leah and Hayley that day. Hayley had recently married. She gleefully stood up, point to her belly and said, "We're expecting our first child." I was so happy for her and her new husband.

They finished eating about the same time I did. I told Leah I'd been sick. I'd only been talking for about 15 seconds when she stopped me. She told me what I needed to do.

She's a gifted, licensed therapist, and her wisdom has always amazed me. I'd gone through months and months of wasted doctor's appointments, with no results. Now, a mere 15 seconds with her, and what she had to say made complete sense.

She told me to meet her at her office in a few days, and she would help me. I know God put me in her path so we could re-connect. It brought me the additional support I needed, and gave Leah the opportunity to bless me, like no one else could.

On the day we met at her office, Leah ran a neurotransmitter test on me. The results supported the leaky gut conclusion, which I'd suspected. It also showed how depleted I was on various neurotransmitters, even though I was heavily dosed on antidepressants. Oddly enough, the results relieved the guilt I'd had about not being able to function.

After receiving my results from Leah, I had her explain them to Jimmy. She described to him how thoroughly depleted my body was of the important amino acids and the various neurotransmitters it needed to function and heal. She vindicated me.

It felt more official now—I was not lazy, or crazy, or just sleeping countless hours because I wanted to. I'd been falling down a dark rabbit-hole of dysfunction because my body was so depleted of necessary nutrients and neurochemicals. Additionally, my thyroid was not functioning properly. I had no physical reserves left. What a relief it was to finally understand why my body and mind couldn't operate properly.

I realized there was an analogy to it. If there is no gas in the car's fuel tank, you won't go anywhere. This is what was happening to my body. My neurochemical tank was close to empty. Theoretically, I was eating food. How did I become so depleted? It turns out, leaky gut was only the beginning of my problems. I was realizing the root of my various issues. This is what I'd wanted from day one.

Another analogy: If you don't pull the weeds out by the roots, they will keep growing out of control and eventually choke out your beautiful garden.

Leah put me on natural supplements—the kind of supplements I'd wanted from the beginning of this horrible ordeal. From there, I improved further.

As I put all the pieces of this crazy puzzle together, I began to experience the angry phase of my journey. No longer angry or guilt-ridden with myself, and not angry at my family or friends. I was developing anger toward my doctors, and the psychiatrist, for not listening, but mostly towards my psychiatrist.

From the very beginning, I'd *asked* for natural ways to heal, without pharmaceuticals. I wanted to find natural ways to help my body do its job. But none of them listened. As it turned out, I somehow instinctively knew the path I needed to heal, but they refused to hear me. It took me a very long time to find someone who could help facilitate my holistic path.

The last straw was near. I knew I could no longer allow my feelings to fester or to bring me down again. Two years' worth of stuffing my frustrations down deep was surfacing. It was time to get it off my chest.

Chapter 12

Enough is Enough

AFTER MY CHANCE encounter with Leah, I finally had the rest of the answers I needed. I maintain it was a Divine appointment. I started my neurotransmitter protocol and regained my inner strength. Next, I got my voice back.

My psychiatrist may have heard my words regarding treatment preferences, but I felt like he never really listened to me. This bothered me—a lot.

He had tried to shut me up about finding the root cause for my illness, and addressing it with alternative solutions. I also knew he'd been lying to me when I asked questions. I had done my own research.

Armed with my newly reclaimed energy, voice, and ability to think, I took advantage of my next appointment to tell him how I really felt.

Like a child's earliest attempts when learning to talk, I blurted out what initially came into my mind. My first words to him were, "You suck!"

Not so professional, I agree. I now realize that a great deal of my fury should have been directed to the healthcare system in general. But the months of frustration had built up inside me to a boiling point. I was furious with him. I felt ignored, and now I was finally able to express it aloud.

I finished my short tirade, "This is me, with a little bit of healthy supplementation, still taking your stupid drugs. Imagine how much better I'll be without them."

It was only the beginning of regaining my voice.

As time went on, I asked him to take me off all the various drugs he had prescribed—piggybacking drugs on top of drugs. As a matter of fact, when one of my new doctors saw the list, he was shocked and dismayed at how many antidepressants I was taking, none of which had worked.

Weeks later, finally drug free and able to really think for myself, my usual sass returned. Nothing would hold me back anymore. The next conversation I had with him opened me up to further healing.

It was early 2015. Although I didn't know it at the time, it was to be my last visit with my psychiatrist. I knew I had to get a few more things off my chest. I've learned you can't fully heal while you steep in anger, resentment, or other negative emotions. You have to clear it out of your life, as soon as you can.

When I arrived for my session, I knew I would convey my disappointment with his services. What I didn't expect was how much I ended up speaking my mind.

I had already told my psychiatrist about the neurotransmitter test I had taken, and a summary of the results. But this time I told him in detail, and showed him my results. The look of disbelief on his face was priceless, but for some reason his surprise frustrated me even more.

I felt the red-hot anger quickly building. It rose upward, from the pit of my stomach. The furious heat singed its way up—through my esophagus. The hot coals of rage finally erupted.

From that point, I couldn't stop. For the next 50 minutes or so, I expressed every thought, every feeling and all the repressed anger I had stuffed down over the many months of so called, "treatment." I lit into him, like I never would have believed possible.

"For more than 18 months I've been sick. I've come here, visit after visit, and you experimented on me with drugs on top of more drugs. I am not an experiment. I am a person with a life full of purpose. I believe everyone you treat should go through this neurotransmitter test. The test gives you the information you need—the exact amount of neurotransmitters a person needs in their body. Why didn't you even know about this?

"Every time I came in for my sessions, you guessed at what to prescribe. I am a life, not a guess. I cannot believe you wasted all these months, guessing at what you thought might work. Not only did you guess and practice on me, but you almost killed me. Did you know that?

"On an earlier visit, I would have killed my self afterward, had I not strongly believed in God. Your concepts of 'alternative treatments' were terrifying. I don't believe you even tried to research what else you might be able to offer me. I paid you for a service you did not do properly. I came here to get help and find the hope I needed, and I did not receive it. I feel as though I've been the one doing all the research. I had to go to the bookstore, which at the time was almost impossible for me. Then I started reading to find out what was wrong."

He, of course, interjected here. He seemed to talk *at* me, as if I worked for him.

"Oh no," I stopped him. "I don't work for you. You work for me. You did not do the job I paid you to do. I am telling you this, not just because I'm so mad about it, but also because I thought you were a 'Christian counselor.' There was no faith here. I never felt any hope from you.

"I tell you this because I want every patient who comes into this office to get what they need from you—faith and hope. You'd better start praying and talking to God, because something is wrong here. It's so wrong in fact, that I am probably the only person who is willing to tell you the truth."

Some people seem to think they cannot truly express their feelings to their healthcare provider because they are doctors. This meant nothing to me. I felt he needed to hear this.

"You have a responsibility," I continued. "When you graduated school, they gave you the requirements you needed to pass your exams. It's your responsibility to continue learning. As science learns more about brain and behavior, you need to expand your knowledge base with them. There is no 'one size fits all' approach."

Believe it or not, I didn't intend to disrespect him. I understand he went through a lot of training to get his degree. I was tired of going to a doctor, not being truly listened to, and not getting the help or answers I needed. I'd felt disrespected, so I suppose I'd lost some respect for him. Additionally, I think he received the brunt of my anger towards all my previous healthcare providers, who were not able to help me find answers.

"God has been speaking to you," I continued, "and you've chosen not to listen. This is why I am here. If you don't start listening, what's coming to your door will be worse. Wake up. God is talking to you."

He finally asked what he could do for me, but I had nothing else to say. Anything from him at that point was too little, too late. I felt he had been a hindrance to my healing, not a help. I haven't seen him since.

I don't pull any punches, and I don't sugar-coat or make it palatable when I'm mad. I was pissed off. I felt most of my illness and suffering could have been resolved months ago. If only he had listened to me, and been open to other treatment options. Even if we had tried them and they failed, at least I would have felt heard. All the signs and symptoms were right in front of him.

When I walked out of his office, I went across the hall to see the therapist I liked. I didn't tell her everything, but I suggested she needed to check on him. I explained that what I said to him was tough for him to hear.

After my visit, I was so spent from expressing all my pent up frustrations, I drove home and went to bed immediately. I was exhausted.

There's a lot of new science out there. Like most physicians, he only focuses on one body part at a time. We must look at everything—the whole body, mind, and spirit. I suppose I can't really fault him completely, since he was not trained in the holistic approach.

Ultimately, his lack of training in alternative practices taught me the importance of taking responsibility for my own health. The integrative and functional model—looking at the entire person—allows us to look at rebalancing all aspects of our well-being. It isn't yet a common practice.

Through the Grace of God, I was guided down the path showing me how to put the puzzle together. I'm grateful for how it eventually all worked out. I now have my life back. It doesn't happen overnight. I am still in the process of healing, but I am on the right track now.

Note: Now that I look back at this part of my life, I realize a few things from a new perspective.

One: God knew by allowing me into this aggravating circumstance, he was offering me what I truly needed. It pushed me into researching and discovering what would work to heal me. He also knew that I would build upon my new information and keep learning more—that I would share my knowledge with others.

Two: As it turns out, one of the reasons why nothing had been working was that I had leaky gut. Things weren't being absorbed properly in the first place. I've now learned that my root cause was an autoimmune disorder called celiac disease. But the tricky thing is—there are three types of celiac: typical/symptomatic, atypical and silent/latent.

The typical, or symptomatic celiac disease, exhibits symptoms of: chronic diarrhea, weight loss, failure to thrive and abdominal pain. But I didn't have those symptoms.

The atypical celiac has a different set of symptoms, that you might not ordinarily associate with the disease. Atypical celiac exhibits symptoms of: anemia, constipation, abnormal liver function, low bone mass, obesity, esophageal reflux, and dyspepsia. This is more in alignment with the type I have. Now that I look back with my current knowledge, it's no surprise that it was initially missed.

The silent, or latent type of celiac—as its name hints—gives no signs for the most part. It has no symptoms and is usually only picked up with a screening.

I firmly believe this health crisis and treatment debacle set me on a new life path. But these lessons were not just for me—they are for everyone I might be able to help in the future.

P.S.—Dude. I still want my money back. Seriously.

Chapter 13

Hindsight is 20/20

HAVE YOU EVER asked yourself, "If I had it to do all over again, what would I do differently?"

It's a great question, especially if you want to learn from how things might have gone wrong. Considering what I've learned from my own health issues, let me share a few insights.

Go to Your Medical Doctor

As a health professional, I have learned it's wise to keep your lines of communication open with your medical doctor. You never know when you might need their perspective on what's happening with your health. Besides, you will probably need the records they've kept on you, for baseline comparison from before you started feeling sick.

I didn't really want to go the western, allopathic medical route. The reason I initially did was it served as my first step in trying to understand what was happening to me. My therapist recommended I have a few tests run, to rule out some of the more serious diagnoses. I respected his suggestion. It was a starting point.

In most cases, your physician will proceed with the allopathic route they know. This is how my journey also began. But after many months of frustration, and prescriptions that seemed to mostly work for others, I felt no relief. You can probably imagine how lost we both felt. If this happens to you, don't lose hope, as there are other avenues to explore.

Merely muting the symptoms with a temporary bandage approach was not enough for me, and it shouldn't be good enough for you either. We need to seek a deeper, more permanent solution, hopefully without all the prescriptions and side effects. I wanted my body to work like it's supposed to. I wanted to heal. That should be the goal for all of us.

It was through the trial and error experience, I learned my main goal had to be finding the root cause of my medical issues. Since most doctors are generally trained to address symptoms, diagnose illness, and prescribe either pharmaceuticals or surgery (great for broken bones or burst appendix), we have to look elsewhere for answers. We need to find a medical practitioner who specializes in functional or integrative medicine.

Please understand something. At this point I don't blame my doctors, or hold any hard feelings toward them. I know they did the best they could with the training they have. But I wanted a more holistic healing approach than what they could offer.

If you find yourself in a similar situation, I'd recommend moving on. Don't waste your time and money with someone who is a bad fit for you. Ask trusted friends for a referral, or go online and look for a functional or integrative medical practitioner. There are plenty of other options available to you.

It took me a while to realize the truth of the adage, "Sometimes if you want a job done right, you have to do it yourself."

I finally realized most mainstream doctors don't have the luxury of time, or the financial initiative to research alternatives or root causes for their patients. Since I didn't have a holistic-health minded practitioner who was trained with this knowledge, the research fell to me. If you cannot find a holistic-minded practitioner, you might need to do the same. Computer search engines become your friend.

It was hard. With what little energy I had, it became my job to find the information and the people with the right approach to help me heal. If you have to, enlist the help of a friend to assist in your research. It's your wellbeing we are talking about here.

Keep track of All Your Lab Results

Remember when I suggested it's wise to keep the lines of communication open with your medical doctor? This is where you can ask for copies of any of your lab work over the past three or four years. You'll need to review your results and look for trends or changes.

It's important to find someone to help you make sense of your results. Occasionally things are missed. Ideally, your doctor catches this. But in reality, it will be up to you to ensure they are double and triple checked. Remember, it's your body. You live in it. You know it better than anyone, and you have the most at stake.

You'll have to take responsibility. Check each level and compare the current results with past results. You'll need to see if there are any deviations. If you don't have access to any such records, then you simply start where you are. Make the best of it.

For optimal results, you'll need to learn what kind of tests you need and ask your doctor to run them. This is not so much telling your doctor what to do, as it is being a participant in your own healing process. If you don't know what lab tests you need, then read, read, and read some more. Research it.

For me, if I had learned more about what tests I needed, I could have healed more quickly. As it was, my first endocrinologist didn't order the full panel of testing and gave me bad information. This happens a lot more often than you'd think it does.

Having only ordered minimal thyroid testing, she ruled my thyroid to be normal. She told me my depression had nothing to do with my thyroid. I learned later, due to the incomplete testing, she had been quite wrong.

It turns out, I have Hashimoto's Thyroiditis, an auto-immune condition. If my first endocrinologist had run the entire panel of correct thyroid testing on me in the first place, she would have seen the problem. Many other people have shared similar experiences. That's why it's so important to learn more about what testing you need.

I understand that the first time around, many times doctors only run a Thyroid Stimulating Hormone test (TSH) and not a complete thyroid panel. This often won't give us the clearest picture of where all the thyroid gland markers are. The complete thyroid panel makes a world of difference, often showing us hidden clues. This helps us see if there are antibodies out of whack, or if various levels don't match a healthy body. You can have some levels be "within normal range," but not be "normal" for you.

Knowing this now makes me shake my head in wonderment. Not only did I suffer longer than necessary, but my new endocrinologist has paid the price for the other doctor's mistake. I now go in, and I mindfully make sure the correct tests are being drawn—even when he says, "We don't usually do this."

I tell him, "I don't care. Humor me and do it anyway."

Always Ask Questions

Before I go to the doctor, I do some research and think up my list of questions. I write them down, and take them with me to my appointment. This way, I won't forget anything, and I can go through them, one by one, with my doctor. I always do this now.

When I was at my sickest point, I could barely speak. My energy was so low I couldn't think straight. Believe me when I tell you, asking for help was not my normal "M.O." But I had no other acceptable choice.

It's hard for someone to speak for you, when they don't fully understand what you're going through, and have no previous medical knowledge. But my husband had to do all the talking and thinking for me. The only thing I could really do was sign my name. That was it. I was broken to a point I would never want anyone to experience.

Question Everything

I'm not like my husband, who was taught never to question a doctor. Maybe the difference for me is I've worked around the medical profession my entire adult life. I've seen some really great doctors, and some not so great. I'm merely saying that as the consumer, you need to do your homework before your visit.

It's important that you educate yourself. Doctors are busy and have a lot on their plate. They can be preoccupied with other things. The more you know going in, the more productive your visit.

When I go to see the doctor, at some time during that appointment, I let them know I am in charge of my health. I tell him or her we need to work as health partners. I ask questions. If I don't like the answers I'm getting, I open a discussion about it.

Don't be afraid to ask plenty of questions, and insist upon understanding what they are talking about. You must realize this is your life and wellbeing you're advocating. And remember, "a little honey helps the medicine go down." So always be nice, and at least it should get you further along working with your doctor.

Be Clear Regarding "Who's the Boss?"

For some reason, most people seem to think their doctor is the boss. Not me. When I visit doctors, I let them know we are partners in my healthcare. I often request specific tests and explain my reasons. Usually, they humor me and I get the answers I need.

Remember, you are in charge of your own health. I say this so you will remember your doctor is supposed to be working for you, and with you. It should be a team approach. It goes both ways. You need to take responsibility for your day-to-day choices.

For this reason, when I was not getting what I needed from my psychiatrist, I finally let him know I'd had enough. If your doctor doesn't meet your needs, you have choices. Have a discussion, and see if things can change. Otherwise move on.

Now that we're done with the basic advice, I suggest the following steps, in any order that's comfortable for you.

Find a Functional or Integrative Medical Provider

This is what I finally did. I eventually found a doctor who was willing to listen, and who was trained in a more holistic approach. Once I found him, he spent time with me and heard my story. He listened intently as I described what happened to me. Then he asked pertinent questions along the way. For the first time, someone was willing to take more than 15 minutes, and listen to everything I had to say. He learned what he needed from me in that process.

If you need to find a functional or integrative medical practitioner in your area, you can do an Internet search for those types of doctors. You can also ask your current doctor, who may know others who practice integrative or functional medicine. You could even ask your friends. I discovered asking suggestions from friends on Facebook can get a great response. There's a growing number of people out there who use integrative or functional medicine practitioners.

Here is another great resource I have used. Not only can you find practicing physicians, but this site is great for learning more about functional medicine.

Visit https://www.functionalmedicine.org

Hire a Health Coach, Trained at Institute for Integrative Nutrition® (IIN®)

Most of my clients have access to insurance and a lot of doctors. But they come to see me because they still have symptoms, which are not going away. They need guidance to implement changes.

IIN® coaches look at all aspects of your life. We go through intense training on many facets of wellness, including 100 different dietary theories. We look at Primary Foods[19], as well as Secondary Foods.

Primary Foods, as you now know, are not what people might think. It's about looking at the other areas of your life, making sure they're balanced. If they're not, take the steps needed to change it. Then everything else gradually starts easing back into balance. These topics go beyond the food we eat, and delve into other important areas of life. When you bring your Circle of Life into balance, multiple aspects of wellness improve. IIN® coaches are trained in an amazing array of additional health and wellness topics.

I decided I wanted more than a just a health coach. I chose to go through the health coach-training program myself. I wanted to learn about the 100 dietary theories, and why they worked for some people or didn't work for others.

This step actually saved my life. Food is the only medicine to which you expose yourself three times a day. According to Ann Wigmore[20], "The food you eat can be either the safest and most powerful form of medicine or the slowest form of poison."

It took me three months of learning and trying out different theories before I discovered the right combination for me.

It was this education on food that started my healing process. It became my first line of defense. You've probably heard, "you are what you eat." This is partly true. But it's also how your body

---

[19] Primary Food(s), and Secondary Food(s): © 2005 Integrative Nutrition, Inc. (used with permission).

[20] Dr. Ann Wigmore, founded the original Hippocrates Health Institute, in Boston, MA, in 1961.

processes what you eat and how (and if) you assimilate your food properly. More accurately, "You are what you absorb." This also happens to pertain to various toxins in your environment.

You can hire an IIN®[21] Coach, but if you want a more in-depth experience, you can enroll in the program. Here is my Institute for Integrative Nutrition® link:

http://geti.in/1zbWHbz

I now have my life back, thanks to IIN®. I can live the life I'm supposed to live. IIN® was my destiny, and it gave me a new purpose. I'm now able to help others. I bring to the table an experience beyond words. I'm living it.

Functional Diagnostic Nutrition® Practitioner

I am not only a graduate of IIN®, I have also become a Certified Functional Diagnostic Nutrition®[22] Practitioner. What does this mean?

I have taken a laboratory course to expand my education on nutritional and functional diagnostics. This means I can speak with a client, ask questions, and gain the information needed to guide them toward their next course of action. That's how I assess which tests are indicated for identifying next steps in their functional healing process.

I can order and send the lab test materials to the client's home. Then I guide them in carrying out the testing and returning of materials to the lab. After that, I review their lab test results and guide them through a next course of action. This is the first move in discovering the root causes to their health issues. My training includes a unique, step-by-step system, called the D.R.E.S.S for Health Success® program.

---

[21] IIN® is © 2005 Integrative Nutrition, Inc. (used with permission).

[22] Functional Diagnostic Nutrition® and D.R.E.S.S for Health Success® are registered trademarks of FDN, Inc. © 2007-2016 FDN, Inc. (used with permission).

This system delves into the five (D.R.E.S.S.®) primary health pillars, identifying "healing opportunities." While each client may need to go about it differently, we always start by looking deeply into the first pillar—a client's Diet. The other pillars we address are Rest, Exercise, Stress reduction, and Supplementation. The FDN materials describe this unique approach as a "scientifically-based, holistically-grounded, repeatedly proven" method that "educates and empowers people to enjoy abundant health—naturally."

I can also work with the client's healthcare practitioner as part of the health team. To learn more about my training in this area, here's my specific FDN link:

https://ua175.isrefer.com/go/CertOptin/a94/

Hindsight tends to be 20/20. These are the steps I would have taken, had I known of these options when I became sick.

Stress was the main culprit in my life. It took me down a road I would never want to go again. As we say in the world of functional medicine, when it came to my health condition, "The gun was loaded, but stress was what pulled the trigger."

The illness I experienced has changed my life, and the direction of my work. I now have my own business, and I'm able to help others who are suffering as I was.

My education is not yet done. As I write here about my journey, I am earning my masters' degree in Human Nutrition and Functional Medicine at the University of Western States. I'm so excited that I can now teach others about the health related issues that break down the body. I can convey it in a way that makes it easy for the layperson to understand.

For more information, please contact me at:

www.holisticdigestivesolutions.com

Chapter 14

Conclusion

THIS MAY BE the conclusion of my book, but it's certainly not the end of my story—it's only the beginning. It can be a new beginning for you as well. Now you can find the health you deserve, and stop chasing your symptoms.

Let me help you find a realistic solution to your health issues, using the outline below, and the resources you'll find in the Appendix.

"You will never know the depths of health, until you lose it." —Unknown

Anyone who's been dealing with multiple health issues understands this. Those who are careless with their lifestyle have yet to learn it.

From my experience, I can recommend taking the following steps:

1. See your current healthcare provider. Retrieve any records and lab results they might have on you over the past three or four years. It's a baseline other providers can use for comparison.

2. If you want to take an alternative approach to heal your entire body (mind & spirit included), then visit the Functional Medicine website and find a practitioner in your area.[23] You'll be seeking a functional or integrative medical practitioner. Also see Appendix for more resources.

3. Hire an Integrative Nutrition® Health Coach. We can be the most beneficial person on your team. We can assist your practitioner by guiding you through any changes they suggest. We will address Primary Foods[24], which in turn will help you with long-range health goals.

4. Find a Functional Diagnostic Nutrition®[25]Practitioner so they can use functional lab work to look deeper. If all your conventional lab work looks good, but you still have symptoms, I would definitely seek their help.

5. Find a functional nutritionist or a practitioner who can look at your dietary and lifestyle habits from a more integrative perspective. They have some incredible training using evidence-based, functional medicine. They work hand in hand with functional medical practitioners, looking at the systems of the body, rather than one body system at a time.

A word (or 50) about the quick recommendations. Please don't let any of these overwhelm or freak you out. Baby-steps, baby. One swap a day, here or there, is a great way to start. Next week—a couple more swaps a day. Awesome. Then, three or four swaps a day by next month, and you're on your way. Keep going.

---

[23] www.Functionalmedicine.org

[24] Primary Food(s), and Secondary Food(s): © 2005 Integrative Nutrition, Inc. (used with permission).

[25] Functional Diagnostic Nutrition® is a registered trademark of FDN, Inc. © 2007-2016 FDN, Inc. (used with permission).

If I could give you a few quick recommendations on food habits, here are the big ones:

1. Eliminate sodas, energy drinks, high-sugar drinks, as well as diet drinks. Instead, swap out drinking lots of lemon water, or just plain water. It's got to be water in order to carry out the toxins and fat cells. The liver and kidneys demand it.

   To figure the proper amount of water to drink, use your weight in pounds, then change that number to ounces and divide by two. Example: If you are 180 pounds, change that to 180 ounces. Divide that by two and it equals 90 ounces of water you should drink every day. You can always add different fruits to your water to liven it up.

2. Start moving your body.[26] Go for walks. They don't have to start out long or fast. Just get out there. Start with five minutes and work your way up. There are also YouTube videos available (for free) which teach you chair yoga and many other exercises appropriate for those who have injuries.

3. Get rid of processed, prepackaged foods. This was one of the first things I did. These foods are loaded with toxic, man-made chemicals, and ingredients that can damage your health.

   Hint: If it has ingredient names that are hard to pronounce, you don't need to be eating it. Also, if it has more than 6 or 8 ingredients, you should most likely get rid of it.

---

[26] I must reiterate here, always consult with your healthcare practitioner, before embarking upon any exercise routines. If you have questions about health concerns and exercise, you can learn more by visiting this web link at MayoClinic.org: http://www.mayoclinic.org/healthy-lifestyle/fitness/in-depth/exercise/art-20047414

4. Eat more vegetables and fruit. Instead of seeing it as getting rid of processed foods, look at it as swapping these healthy, nutritious, nutrient-dense foods for the old, health-stealing, regular stuff. Remember, food can either cause or heal disease. Ideally make 50% of your plate full of vegetables and fruits.

   Eventually, your tastes will change, and you won't miss the old offenders. You will be amazed when you go this route. Once you realize you have the control, it becomes a no brainer.

   You probably won't need a doctor to approve of those previous 3 steps. They are wise things to do getting started on your path back to health.

   But the next step, is one you should probably talk about with your healthcare provider.

5. Look into doing an elimination diet if you have chronic health conditions. Please visit my website[27] to learn more about different types of elimination diets, and information regarding the various health conditions which are helped with such diets.

6. Find a doctor who is willing to work *with* you, towards your health goals. Make them part of your wellness team.

---

[27] www.holisticdigestivesolutions.com

Appendix

Information and Resources for Your Ongoing Transformation

Websites:

My website: www.holisticdigestivesolutions.com

Learn more about the Joe Cross reboot:
www.rebootwithjoe.com

Find a functional health practitioner:
www.functionalmedicine.org

Get the list for the Dirty Dozen and the Clean 15:
www.ewg.org/foodnews/index.php)

Find local (CSAs) community supported agriculture:
www.localharvest.org/csa/

Learn more about superfoods, with David Wolfe:
http://www.davidwolfe.com/

Vitamix® emulsifying blenders:
https://www.vitamix.com/Home

NutriBullet® (blenders) Nutrient Extractors (David Wolfe uses them)
https://nutribullet.com/

Blendtec® emulsifying blenders:
http://www.blendtec.com/blenders

Movies/Documentaries:

Fat, Sick and Nearly Dead

Fat, Sick and Nearly Dead 2

Fed Up

Hungry for Change

FOOD, Inc.

Vegucated

Education:

Institute for Integrative Nutrition® link here:
http://geti.in/1zbWHbz

Functional Diagnostic Nutrition®
https://ua175.isrefer.com/go/CertOptin/a94/

University of Western States http://www.uws.edu

Books: (Note—Check my website for a more in-depth list of books that I keep adding.) www.holisticdigestivesolutions.com)

About Thyroid:

Why Do I Still Have Thyroid Symptoms? When My Lab Tests Are Normal
by Datis Kharrazian
(This is one of the best books I have read. It's easy to understand and great for the average layperson.)

Hashimoto's Thyroiditis: Lifestyle Interventions for Finding and Treating the Root Cause
by Izabella Wentz PharmD (This book is a little more science based.)

About Brain:

The UltraMind Solution,
 by Dr. Mark Hyman, MD

Why Isn't My Brain Working?: A Revolutionary Understanding of Brain Decline and Effective Strategies to Recover Your Brain's Health,
by Datis Kharrazian

About Candida:

The Body Ecology Diet,
by Donna Gates

Living Candida-Free: 100 Recipes and a 3-Stage Program to Restore Your Health and Vitality media matrix,
by Ricki Heller& Andrea Nakayama

About Juicing:

The Reboot with Joe Juice Diet,
by Joe Cross

About the Author:

Karen Thomas is a Registered Dental Hygienist, a Certified 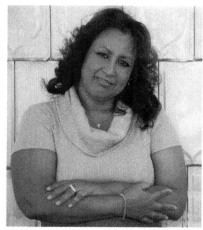 Functional Diagnostic Nutrition® Practitioner (FDN-P), a Certified Integrative Nutrition® Health Coach, an Author, and she is also an Educator and Motivational Speaker.

She received her AS in Dental Hygiene from Palm Beach State College in Lake Worth, Florida. Then she received her BS in Dental Hygiene from the University of North Carolina, at Chapel Hill. Karen received her health coach training from the Institute for Integrative Nutrition®, in New York City, NY. She received her FDN-P training from Functional Diagnostic Nutrition®, in Poway, California.

She's currently working toward her Master's degree in Human Nutrition and Functional Medicine, at the University of Western States, in Portland, Oregon.

Karen personally understands the struggles of chronic illness. It's why she works with people who are stressed, depressed, fatigued and suffering chronic health conditions. Clients describe her as motivating, inspiring, and hopeful. For more information on Karen or to learn more about functional nutrition, please visit her website:

www.holisticdigestivesolutions.com.

Made in the USA
Middletown, DE
27 January 2022

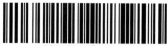

59753215R00068